SMALL ANIMAL ANAESTHESIA
THE INCREASED-RISK PATIENT

PATRICIA BURKE, D.V.M.

SMALL ANIMAL ANAESTHESIA
THE INCREASED-RISK PATIENT

Edited by

P. G. C. BEDFORD, BVetMed, PhD, FRCVS, DVOphthal
University Reader in Veterinary Ophthalmology,
Royal Veterinary College, University of London

Baillière Tindall Limited
London Philadelphia Toronto Sydney Tokyo

This book is printed on acid-free paper

Baillière Tindall   24–28 Oval Road
W. B. Saunders   London NW1 7DX, England

The Curtis Center, Independence Square West
Philadelphia, PA 19106–3399, USA

55 Horner Avenue
Toronto, Ontario M8Z 4X6, Canada

Harcourt Brace Jovanovich (Australia) Pty Ltd
30–52 Smidmore Street,
Marrickville, NSW 2204, Australia

Harcourt Brace Jovanovich Japan Inc.
Ichibancho Central Building, 22–1 Ichibancho
Chiyoda-ku. Tokyo 102, Japan

© 1991 Baillière Tindall

A catalogue record for this book is available
from the British Library

ISBN 0-7020 1501-6

Typeset by Cambridge Composing (UK) Ltd, Cambridge
Printed in Great Britain by Mackays of Chatham PLC, Chatham, Kent

Contents

The contributors

Nicholas H. Dodman graduated from the University of Glasgow Veterinary School in 1970. From 1970 to 1971 he completed a surgical internship at the same school and then went into general practice for a short while. In 1972 Mr Dodman was appointed lecturer in surgery at the Glasgow Veterinary School where he was employed in that capacity until 1981. In 1975 he obtained a DVA by examination. From 1981 to date Mr Dodman has worked at Tufts University School of Veterinary Medicine in Massachusetts. He obtained diplomate status of the American College of Veterinary Anesthesiologists in 1982 and is currently an Associate Professor and Chief of the Anesthesia Service at Tufts Veterinary School.

Michael H. Court received his BVSc degree from the University of Queensland School of Veterinary Science in 1981. He then enrolled in the small animal internship programme at the University of Sydney and, in 1982, he received a Diploma in Veterinary Clinical Studies. In 1983, Mr Court entered the veterinary anaesthesia residency programme at Tufts University and subsequently achieved diplomate status (by examination) of the American College of Veterinary Anesthesiologists in 1987. Mr Court is currently an Assistant Professor in the Anesthesia Section of the Department of Surgery at Tufts University.

Wendy M. Norman graduated from the University of Queensland School of Veterinary Science in 1981. Since then she has completed a small animal internship in anaesthesia at the University of Sydney and a veterinary anaesthesia residency programme at Tufts University. Ms Norman is now Assistant Professor of Anesthesiology in the Department of Large Animal Clinical Sciences at the University of Florida in Gainesville, Florida.

David Seeler received his DVM degree from the Ontario Veterinary College in 1978 and completed an internship in anaesthesiology at

Small animal anaesthesia

the same institution the following year. After receiving a Master of Science degree from the University of Guelph, he completed a residency programme in anaesthesia at the University of Illinois. In 1983, he accepted a faculty position at the Tufts University School of Veterinary Medicine, and in 1984, he became a diplomate of the American College of Veterinary Anesthesiologists. He is also a member of the New York Academy of Sciences. Dr Seeler is currently an Associate Professor of Anaesthesiology in the Department of Companion Animals at the Atlantic Veterinary College, Prince Edward Island, Canada.

Leslie L. Fikes, Assistant Professor in Surgery at the Tufts University School of Veterinary Medicine, contributed to the chapter on anaesthesia for patients with neuromuscular disease.

Foreword

The development of improved anaesthetic techniques and the emergence of new anaesthetic agents has meant that the prognosis for the small animal patient undergoing surgery has improved considerably over recent years. The facility of general anaesthesia is now recognized as an essential part of clinical service work, and the development of expertise in practice has allowed the range of treatment posssible to expand very considerably. Anaesthesia has always involved some risk to the patient, but that risk may be increased in certain disease situations. In this text, Dr Dodman and his associates have examined several areas of increased risk in terms of specific anaesthetic considerations and requirements, and their recommendations are interpreted as sound practical advice.

1

Protocol for general anaesthesia in small animal patients

General anaesthesia is required for a variety of surgical and diagnostic procedures in small animal practice. Although anaesthetic mishaps occur occasionally, their incidence can be minimized by the adoption of a protocol designed to ensure the appropriate level of preoperative, intraoperative and postoperative care. An anaesthetic protocol will provide guidelines which enable the veterinary surgeon to:

1. Ensure adequate preanaesthetic preparation.
2. Identify poor risk patients prior to anaesthesia.
3. Standardize techniques in order to minimize technical error.
4. Provide optimum intraoperative supportive therapy.
5. Monitor patients and assist in the early detection of potential complications.
6. Ensure adequate postoperative care.

Individuals vary in their opinion as to what constitutes safe anaesthetic practice. It is generally agreed, however, that the adoption of a scheme which increases patient care will minimize the incidence of perioperative complications.

PREANAESTHETIC EVALUATION AND PREPARATION

The physical examination of a surgical patient is the first step in determining the potential anaesthetic risk. All animals, even those which are young and apparently healthy, should have a physical examination performed prior to anaesthesia. The evaluation of cardiopulmonary, hepatic and renal function is of particular importance at this time. When the initial examination reveals an abnormality, a more detailed investigation is warranted. This often involves the use of ancillary diagnostic tests.

Table 1. Classification of patient's physical status*

Category	Physical condition	Examples of possible situations
Class I Minimal risk	Normal healthy animal No underlying disease	Ovariohysterectomy, castration, declawing operation, hip dysplasia radiograph
Class II Slight risk	Animals with slight to mild systemic disturbances Animal able to compensate No clinical signs of disease	Neonate or geriatric animals, obesity, fracture without shock, mild diabetes, compensating heart or kidney disease
Class III Moderate risk	Animals with moderate systemic disease or disturbances Mild clinical signs	Anaemia, anorexia, moderate dehydration, low-grade kidney disease, low-grade heart murmur or cardiac disease, moderate fever
Class IV High risk	Animals with pre-existing systemic disease or disturbances of a severe nature	Severe dehydration, shock, anaemia, uraemia or toxaemia, high fever, uncompensated heart disease, diabetes or pulmonary disease
Class V Grave risk	Surgery often performed in desperation on animals with life-threatening systemic disease or disturbances not often correctable by an operation. Includes all moribund animals not expected to survive 24 h. Little need for general anaesthesia as the moribund state renders the animal oblivious to pain	Advanced cases of heart, kidney, liver, lung or endocrine disease, profound shock, major head injury, severe trauma, pulmonary embolus

* An 'E' is added to the classification if the procedure is of an emergency nature.

The findings of the examination, along with the clinical history, should enable the anaesthetist to evaluate the anaesthetic risk to the patient. Table 1 is a classification of anaesthetic risk. The majority of patients are normally in excellent or good health. These patients, identified as class I or class II, can be safely anaesthetized using standard techniques. Patients in class III often need to be

Table 2. Laboratory tests required begore general anaesthesia

Risk status	Less than 6 years	Over 6 years
Class I and II	PCV, TP, BUN	CBC, UA, BUN
Class III	CBC, UA, BUN	CBC, UA, BUN, ALT, SG
Class IV and V	CBC, UA, CP	CBC, UA, CP

PCV	packed cell volume.	UA	urinalysis.
TP	total serum protein.	CP	serum chemistry profile.
BUN	blood urea nitrogen.	ALT	alanine transaminase (SGPT).
CBC	complete blood count.	SG	serum glucose.

stabilized prior to anaesthesia and different techniques may be indicated. Class IV and V patients require intensive physiological support and monitoring throughout the anaesthetic period. In all instances good anaesthetic practice will decrease perianaesthetic morbidity and mortality.

Routine screening tests are recommended to reduce the possibility of anaesthetizing a patient with subclinical disease. A list of appropriate tests is given in Table 2. Most of these tests can easily be performed in a practice laboratory.

A form similar to the one illustrated in Fig. 1 can be used to standardize the preanaesthetic evaluation procedure. A checklist like this is particularly valuable when more than one person is contributing to the preparation of the patient. The anaesthetic record (Fig. 2) should be started prior to or at the time of premedication. Agents used for premedication, induction, and maintenance of anaesthesia, in addition to their dose rates and routes of administration, should be recorded on this form.

Food should be withheld from the healthy patient for 8 to 12 h prior to the induction of anaesthesia (Booth and McDonald, 1982). In very young animals, a shorter period of fasting has been recommended (Short and Brunson, 1978). Prolonged fasting depletes liver glycogen reserves and renders the animal less capable of withstanding the stress of surgery and anaesthesia. Fluids need only be withheld for approximately 2 h. Water deprivation for excessive periods of time is undesirable since it can lead to dehydration and hypovolaemia.

PREMEDICATION

Atropine is used preoperatively for its anti-sialogogue and vago-lytic effects. While atropine may be used routinely prior to anaes-thesia, administration only when specifically indicated is advised. This is because atropine can cause autonomic imbalance which

Purpose of Anaesthesia:	Patient Data: Owner's Name Address
Primary Condition:	Telephone Number Patient's Name Age
Concurrent Disease(s):	Breed Sex Body Weight

History/Physical/Laboratory Exam Data

1. T_____   P_____   R_____

2. Cardiovascular: PCV_____   TP_____
    Memb. Colour:_____   CRT_____
    Auscultation:_____
    ECG taken:_____Results:_____

3. Respiratory: Auscultation

    _____

4. Thoracic Radiographs:_____Date:_____

    Results:_____

5. Serum Chemistries:
    BUN:_____   AST:_____
     G:_____   Alk. Phos.:_____
    Other:_____

6. Urinalysis
    Colour:_____   Specific Gravity:_____
       pH:_____   Protein:_____
    Glucose:_____   Cells:_____
    Other:_____

7. Current Medications and/or Prior Anaesthetics

    _____

Physical Status:_____

Anaesthetic Problems:_____

Anaesthetic Plan:_____

Fig. 1   Preanaesthetic evaluation form.

will predispose the patient to dangerous sympathetic-mediated cardiac dysrhythmias (Muir, 1978). The resultant tachycardia is also undesirable when the resting heart rate is high. If an anticholinergic effect is required when the resting heart rate is high, glycopyrronium (glycopyrrolate) is more suitable because it has

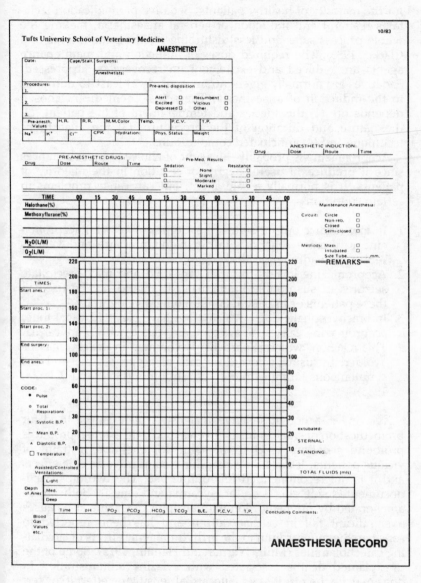

Fig. 2 Anaesthesia record form.

less chronotropic action. Finally, it should be remembered that in certain circumstances low doses of atropine may result in centrally-induced bradycardia and hypotension.

The use of sedative premedicant drugs is highly recommended

for the majority of healthy patients. Sedative premedication facilitates restraint and induction of general anaesthesia, making the whole process safer and less disturbing for the patient (Hall and Clarke, 1983). The required doses of induction and maintenance agents are reduced and excitement on recovery is suppressed. Sedatives are normally given intramuscularly at least 15 min prior to the induction of anaesthesia. The actual premedicant chosen depends on: (1) the species and temperament of the patient, (2) the nature and duration of the procedure, (3) the anaesthetic technique and (4) anticipated complications.

Acepromazine is probably the agent of choice in most instances since it produces a useful degree of sedation in the majority of patients. It is normally a safe agent, but can cause problems in certain conditions:

1. In low cardiac output states (most types of 'shock') acepromazine can cause a serious fall in blood pressure and venous return by α-adrenergic blockade.
2. Acepromazine lowers the ictal threshold and may precipitate seizures in susceptible individuals. It should not be used in these patients or in patients undergoing myelography.
3. In brachycephalic dogs, which often have elevated vagal tone, acepromazine can cause syncope associated with bradycardia. This reaction, which is particularly common in Boxers, may be avoided by using a low dose rate of acepromazine and the simultaneous administration of atropine (Hall and Clarke, 1983).

Xylazine is a potent sedative-analgesic which can be used for premedication of small animals. Even at a low dose rate it produces profound sedation which is of value for chemical restraint of vicious patients. It does, however, have some adverse side effects and it is not recommended for routine use. The two most well-documented side effects are bradycardia and emesis. Both can be ameliorated by premedication with atropine. Xylazine also causes a significant fall in cardiac output and has been reported to sensitize the myocardium to the arrhythmogenic effects of circulating catecholamines (Muir, Werner and Hamlin, 1975). Some of the unexplained deaths associated with xylazine administration in dogs may be the result of its myocardial sensitizing effect (Sawyer, 1982). Medetomidine, a compound with a similar action to xylazine, but with longer duration of action, has become available recently. Both xylazine and medetomidine can be reversed with a specific antagonist, atipamezole, if a quick recovery is desired or if an adverse reaction occurs.

Narcotic analgesics are occasionally given to dogs and cats

Table 3. Comparison of induction agents

	Thiopentone	Methohexitone	Saffan	Ketamine
Intravenous				
dose rate (a) Unpremedicated	16–25	8–10	6–9	5–10
mg kg⁻¹ (b) Premedicated	8–12	4–6	3–5	5–10
Cardiovascular depression	Moderate	Moderate	Mild	Very little
Respiratory depression	Moderate	Moderate	Mild	Very little
Adverse effects	Perivascular irritancy	Excitement	Histamine release	Convulsions in the dog ?hallucination
Species in which used	Dog or cat	Dog or cat	Cat	Cat
Length of recovery	Moderate	Rapid	Rapid	Slow
Therapeutic safety	Fair	Fair	Good	Good

preoperatively for their sedative or analgesic effects. They are probably best administered in combination with a neuroleptic drug as the two agents will potentiate each other. Atropine should also be administered to prevent the inevitable narcotic-induced bradycardia. Proprietary neuroleptanalgesic combinations such as Hypnorm (fentanyl and fluanisone, Janssen Pharmaceutica) or Immobilon (etorphine and methotrimeprazine, Reckitt and Colman) can also be used for preoperative sedation. A safety feature of these combinations is that the narcotic analgesic component can be reversed at any time with a specific antagonist such as naloxone. Suggested dose rates of agents used for premedication are listed in Appendix I.

INDUCTION

Smooth atraumatic inductions are essential in order to provide good anaesthetic care for the patient. Table 3 compares the four most commonly used induction agents. Thiopentone is recommended as the agent of choice in dogs. A standard strength of thiopentone solution should be used on all occasions to avoid confusion. A 2.5% solution is advisable. This concentration is considerably less irritant to the tissues than a 5% solution and will be associated with a lower incidence of perivascular sloughs (Soma, 1971). If thiopentone is inadvertently injected perivascularly, then lignocaine (lidocaine) should be used to infiltrate the area. This precipitates and dilutes the perivascular thiopentone. Additional dilution with normal saline may be useful.

Methohexitone can also be used for the induction of anaesthesia in dogs and cats. It has the great advantage of being rapidly metabolized so that full recovery from its effects is quick. It should be used for induction of anaesthesia in out-patients and in animals expected to have a prolonged recovery following thiopentone. The latter group would include immature animals up to four months of age, geriatric animals, sighthounds and animals with impaired hepatic function. Unfortunately, methohexitone has excitatory side effects and because of this, is more difficult to use successfully. Dogs and cats induced with methohexitone should normally be premedicated with a sedative drug to minimize induction excitement. Underdosage may result in excitement while a relative or absolute overdose will cause apnoea. In either case, the transition from induction to inhalational maintenance can be difficult. Recovery from methohexitone may also be associated with excitement.

In dogs, induction agents are best administered via an intravenous catheter. The catheter should remain in place throughout the period of anaesthesia and into the recovery period. This will minimize accidental perivascular injections and facilitate the intraoperative and postoperative administration of fluids and drugs. As the placement of intravenous catheters is difficult in conscious cats, it is often only possible to insert the catheters after the induction of anaesthesia.

In cats, either Saffan (alphaxalone/alphadolone) or thiopentone is commonly used for induction of anaesthesia (Dodman, 1977). Saffan appears to be the agent of choice. The advantages of Saffan include its high therapeutic index, convenient duration of action, lack of accumulation, minimal physiological depression, and little or no tissue irritancy (Child *et al.*, 1971). Problems (erythema, oedema and cyanosis), probably associated with histamine release induced by the vehicle, have been reported (Dodman, 1980); however, some practitioners feel that the advantages of Saffan probably outweigh the potential problems. Alternative vehicles are being researched currently, and future developments may render Saffan safe for use in other species too.

Ketamine is used to induce anaesthesia in cats in some practices. It can be administered either intravenously, subcutaneously or intramuscularly. The type of anaesthesia produced has been described as 'dissociative'. The eyes remain open, pharyngeal and laryngeal reflexes persist, and muscle tone and salivation are increased. Ketamine can be used as the sole anaesthetic for minor procedures, but full recovery from its effects may take several hours. It should not be used alone for major surgery including laparotomy, as visceral analgesia is incomplete at the advocated dosage. (The dose rates of the commonly used intravenous induction agents are listed in Appendix I.)

Animals less than two months of age should be induced with an inhalational agent. Owing to their body composition and immature metabolism, these animals have a reduced ability to deal with drugs which rely on either redistribution or metabolism to terminate their action. This can result in a considerable delay in recovery from their effects. When a face mask is used for inhalation induction, a bland eye ointment should be instilled into the conjunctival sacs to protect the eyes.

A lubricated endotracheal tube of appropriate diameter should be inserted immediately after the induction of anaesthesia in all but the shortest of anaesthetics. In cats, a lignocaine spray should be used to desensitize the larynx and upper airway prior to intubation. Stilettes are useful to keep the endotracheal tube stiff, but if used, should not protrude past the end of the tube. Forcing a tube through a closed glottis is to be discouraged. The tube should not protrude for more than 1 inch in front of the incisor teeth and its tip should come to lie midway between the larynx and the thoracic inlet. These provisions will ensure that dead space is kept to a minimum and that endobronchial intubation is not performed inadvertently. Endotracheal tubes with high volume, low pressure cuffs are generally recommended in canine anaesthesia. Cuffs should only be inflated to the point where they prevent the escape of air around the tube when a minimal pressure (5 to 10 cmH$_2$O) is applied to the system. Non-cuffed tubes are recommended for use in cats. Most cats will require a 4.5 to 5.0 mm internal diameter endotracheal tube. All endotracheal tubes should be secured with one inch gauze to prevent accidental extubation. When it has not been done previously, a bland eye ointment should be applied to the eyes at this time.

MAINTENANCE OF ANAESTHESIA

Maintenance of general anaesthesia with thiobarbiturates for anything but the shortest procedures cannot be condoned. Continuous administration of these agents will result in lengthy and unpleasant recoveries. Maintenance of anaesthesia in cats by the intermittent injection (or constant infusion) of Saffan is acceptable. The steroid combination is rapidly metabolized by the liver and is therefore non-cumulative (Child *et al.*, 1971).

In general, the patient should be connected to an anaesthetic machine as soon as possible after induction of anaesthesia for maintenance with inhalational agents. The most popular inhalational agent at this time is halothane. A 1 to 2% inspired vapour concentration (in oxygen) is sufficient for most procedures. If 60 to 70% nitrous oxide is used in background mixture then the inspired halothane concentration may be reduced by 22% (De Young and Sawyer, 1980). Isoflurane, an inhalational agent with a similar

Table 4. Scheme for selection of breathing circuits

Body weight	Circuit	Fresh gas flow ml kg^{-1} min^{-1}	Advantages	Disadvantages
Less than 7 kg wt	T-piece Magill Bain (semi-closed)	600 300 130	Precise control of inspired concentration Minimal resistance to flow	High flows make systems expensive to operate
More than 7 kg wt	To and fro or circle absorber system (closed or semi-closed)	6–8 (closed) Up to 100 (semi-closed)	Both circuits make efficient use of fresh gas flow and are therefore inexpensive to operate	Less control over inspired concentration Greater resistance to breathing

potency to halothane, is rapidly gaining popularity as it has several advantages to offer over halothane. Its flexibility, related to its low blood : gas solubility, relative resistance to metabolism (hence minimal toxicity) and lack of myocardial sensitization to the arrhythmogenic effects of adrenaline are some of the advantages to be gained from its use. Whatever agent is selected to maintain anaesthesia, it should be administered by the appropriate breathing circuit (Table 4).

Intravenous fluids should be administered to all animals under general anaesthesia. The use of either normal saline, Ringer's solution or lactated Ringer's solution is satisfactory for this purpose. A rate of infusion of 5 to 10 ml kg^{-1} h^{-1} is adequate in most circumstances. Blood loss of less than 20% of the total blood volume may be replaced using a balanced electrolyte solution. The volume of the electrolyte solution administered is two to three times the volume of the blood lost. Losses greater than 20% should be replaced with whole blood.

All animals should be placed on a heating pad or circulating hot water blanket during anaesthesia to help prevent hypothermia. Hypothermia is associated with a decreased anaesthetic requirement and causes disturbances in most of the patient's physiological processes. The anaesthetic requirement of halothane decreases by 5% per °C drop in core body temperature (Eger, 1984). At 28 °C, the anaesthetic requirement is decreased by 50%. If hypothermia develops and the reduction in anaesthetic requirement is not appreciated by the anaesthetist, overdosage will result. Body temperature below 33 °C will result in bradycardia, unresponsive to atropine, which is best treated with a sympathomimetic agent.

It is most important that all anaesthetized patients are monitored by a trained individual. This is probably the single most important factor in preventing anaesthetic complications. The following parameters should be monitored on a routine basis:

1. Heart rate (use an oesophageal stethoscope).
2. Respiratory rate and depth.
3. Capillary refill time.
4. Colour of mucous membranes.
5. ECG (on oscilloscope).
6. Drugs given during anaesthesia.
7. Rectal temperature.
8. Depth of anaesthesia.

All of the above parameters should be recorded on the anaesthetic record with a maximum time lapse of 5 to 10 min between readings. The use of an ECG in routine cases may seem overly cautious to those not familiar with this form of monitoring; however, it will provide valuable information in the emergency situation. In the extreme case of cardiac arrest it is impossible to treat the condition appropriately unless it is known whether one is dealing with asystole, fibrillation or electromechanical dissociation.

RECOVERY

The patient should be allowed to breathe oxygen for as long as possible after the anaesthetic is discontinued. This offsets the cardiopulmonary depressant effects of the anaesthetic and the increased oxygen consumption caused by shivering. Keeping the patient connected to a properly scavenged breathing circuit during recovery also minimizes operating room pollution. Other measures to reduce operating room pollution are listed in Appendix II.

Endotracheal tubes should be de-cuffed on exit from the surgery. This will help minimize the time during which the tracheal mucosa is compressed and its blood flow compromised by the inflated cuff. As the tube is de-cuffed, the animal should have its lungs inflated so that any material which has accumulated above the cuff is blown into the pharynx. The endotracheal tube should be withdrawn only after the animal has regained control of its laryngeal and pharyngeal reflexes. Withdrawal of the tube should be at the end of inspiration so that expiration or a cough are the only possible respiratory manoeuvres.

All animals are hypothermic to some extent following inhalational anaesthesia. This is because of increased heat loss and decreased heat production during anaesthesia (Waterman, 1975). Warming blankets and/or heat lamps should be available for animals in the recovery area to prevent further heat loss and assist in rewarming. This is particularly important for animals weighing less than 10 kg. The return to consciousness seems to be faster and less stressful when serious falls in body temperature are avoided (Dodman and Brito-Babapulle, 1979).

It is important to continue administering fluids in the recovery period following prolonged procedures or when a protracted recovery is anticipated. If necessary, these fluids should be warmed.

The alleviation of postoperative pain should be a prime concern. This is particularly important when painful orthopaedic or thoracic procedures have been performed. In some cases, postoperative pain can be prevented temporarily by blocking the appropriate regional nerves with a local anaesthetic. The use of the intercostal nerve block following thoracotomy or brachial plexus block following forelimb amputation provides examples of the postoperative application of regional nerve block techniques. When bupivacaine is the local anaesthetic used, pain relief of several hours' duration can be achieved. If the operative site is such that a regional nerve block technique cannot be applied, then the systemic adminis-tration of an opioid agent will provide significant pain relief. Morphine, butorphanol and buprenorphine are examples of opioid agents with a sufficiently long duration of action to provide a useful period of postsurgical analgesia in dogs and cats. Opioid mu receptor agonists such as morphine, however, should be used only at appropriate (low) dosages in cats because of their propen-sity for opioid-induced excitement. Another highly effective way of producing opioid-mediated analgesia is to administer preserva-tive-free preparations of the drugs epidurally. The analgesia pro-duced in this way is particularly long lasting.

All animals should be inspected at regular intervals during the recovery period and have their temperature, pulse and respiration monitored. This will help to prevent postoperative complications, just as monitoring during the operation helps to prevent intraoper-ative complications.

CONCLUSION

The use of a standard, well-conceived anaesthetic protocol in small animal practice will result in improved patient care. A protocol such as the one described, when followed faithfully, will ensure smooth, rapid and atraumatic techniques with minimal stress and risk to the patient.

REFERENCES

Booth, N. H. and McDonald, L. E. (1982). In *Veterinary Pharmacology and Therapeutics*, p. 156, 5th edn. Ames: The Iowa State University Press.

Child, K. J., Currie, J. P., Davis, B., Dodds, M. G., Pearce, D. A. and Twissell, D. J. (1971). *British Journal of Anaesthesia* **43**, 2.

Dodman, N. H. (1977). *Journal of Small Animal Practice* **18**, 653.

Dodman, N. H. (1980). *Veterinary Record* **107**, 481.

Dodman, N. H. and Brito-Babapulle, L. A. P. (1979). *Proceedings of the Association of Veterinary Anaesthetists of Great Britain and Ireland* **No. 8**, 141.

DeYoung, D. J. and Sawyer, D. C. (1980). *Journal of the American Animal Hospital Association* **16**, 125.

Eger, E. I. (1984). In *Anaesthetic Uptake and Action*, p. 11. Baltimore: Williams and Wilkins.

Hall, L. W. and Clarke, K. W. (1983). In *Veterinary Anaesthesia*, p. 70 and 307, 8th edn. London: Baillière Tindall.

Muir, W. W. (1978). *Journal of the American Veterinary Medical Association* **172**(8), 917.

Muir, W. W., Werner, L. L. and Hamlin, R. L. (1975). *American Journal of Veterinary Research* **36**, 1299.

Sawyer, D. C. (1982). In *The Practice of Small Animal Anesthesia*, p. 9. Philadelphia: W. B. Saunders Company.

Short, C. E. and Brunson, D. B. (1978). *Cornell Veterinarian* **68**, 9.

Soma, L. R. (1971). In *Textbook of Veterinary Anesthesia*, p. 275. Baltimore: The Williams and Wilkins Company.

Waterman, A. E. (1975). *Veterinary Record* **96**, 308.

APPENDIX I

Suggested dose rates of anaesthetic agents

Agent	Dose mg kg^{-1}	Route
Acepromazine	0.05–0.10	i.m.
Atropine	0.02–0.06	i.m., i.v.
Butorphanol	0.05–0.1	i.m.
Flunixin	0.75–1.25	i.m.
Glycopyrronium (glycopyrrolate)	0.005–0.01	i.m., i.v.
Hypnorm	0.5 ml kg^{-1}	i.m.
Immobilon	0.1 ml kg^{-1}	i.m.
	0.05 ml kg^{-1}	i.v.
Ketamine	15–40	i.m.
	4–8	i.v.
Methohexitone	4–6*	i.v.
Naloxone	0.006–0.04	i.v.
Pethidine	3–8	i.m.
Saffan	6–9	i.v.
Thiopentone	8–10*	i.v.
Xylazine	0.5–2	i.m.
Medetomodine	0.04	i.m.

* Following sedative premedication.

APPENDIX II. Methods of reducing the level of waste anaesthetic gases in the operating room

1. The installation of an effective scavenging system is essential in reducing trace gas levels in the operating room(s).
2. Anaesthesia machines and their scavenging systems should routinely undergo servicing at regular intervals by a manufacturer's representative to avoid leaks (in-house monitoring is also necessary to ensure that leakage is minimized).
3. Work practices should be modified if necessary—staff monitoring anaesthetics should be trained to avoid practices which lead to high levels of waste gases, e.g. avoid turning on anaesthetic gases until the endotracheal tube is connected to the circuit, exercise care in filling vaporizers, etc.
4. Some thought should be given to the ventilation system of the premises. Ventilation systems of the recirculatory type will cause cross-contamination of several rooms if one room becomes contaminated.
5. Levels of anaesthetic gases should be measured quarterly in the operating room.
6. Anaesthesia personnel should receive periodic reminders that their

efforts are the key to reducing not only their own exposure but also that of their co-workers.

7. A communication should be circulated annually to exposed personnel.

Adapted from: Lecky, J. H. (1981). *Waste Anesthetic Gases in Operating Room Air: a Suggested Program to Reduce Personnel Exposure*. Park Ridge, Illinois: American Society of Anesthesiologists.

2

Anaesthesia for geriatric patients

The transition from middle to old age is a gradual process, and consequently any definition of the start of old age is necessarily arbitrary. Even if a specific age was defined above which dogs and cats were regarded as geriatric, it would not be particularly useful because there are large differences in life expectancy between species, breeds and individuals. For the purpose of this article, the authors suggest that animals be considered as aged when they have completed 75% to 80% of their anticipated life span. An indication of the anticipated life spans of dogs and cats is provided by Bronson (1981, 1982).

Some of the pathophysiological alterations in older animals are the result of the ageing process and are normal degenerative changes. Other changes may result from the progression of chronic disease processes. In the following account, the pathophysiological changes in the major organ systems associated with ageing are described. The impact of these changes on the anaesthetic management of the geriatric small animal patient is discussed.

AGE-RELATED CHANGES IN THE MAJOR ORGAN SYSTEMS

Central nervous system

One of the most apparent signs of ageing in humans and animals is a progressive decline in central nervous system activity. The structure–function relationship in the central nervous system is still far from clear, so it is dangerous to draw too many conclusions regarding function from anatomical or histological changes. It is

Modified with permission from: Dodman, N. H., Seeler, D. C. and Court, M. H. (1984). Aging changes in the geriatric dog and their impact on anesthesia. *The Compendium on Continuing Education for the Practicing Veterinarian (Small Animal)* **6**, 1106.

interesting to note, however, that brain weight has been shown to decrease with age in humans, primarily because of atrophic changes in neurons in the cerebral hemispheres. It is also note-worthy that there are age-related changes in central nerve conduction in humans (Miller, 1981). In addition, there is decreased production and increased destruction of central neurotransmitters (Owens, 1983). An age-related reduction in dose requirement of injectable and inhalational anaesthetics has been demonstrated in people (Muravchick and Mandel, 1982; Eger, 1974). It may be conjectured that less anaesthetic would be needed in older animals.

In addition to the decline of central nervous function with age, the peripheral nerves and neuromuscular junction deteriorate. Coordination is often impaired because of decreased conduction velocity in peripheral nerves (Janis, 1979; Swallow, 1973). The neuromuscular junction also degenerates and the number of receptors on the postsynaptic membrane decreases, although receptor supersensitivity develops in the remaining receptors (Miller, 1981). Prolonged action of muscle relaxants should be anticipated in the elderly.

Geriatric dogs and cats suffer from hearing loss or have some vision impairment. Because of this, they can be startled easily and should be approached carefully. Constant reassurance is necessary to minimize stress, especially when the animal is already apprehensive because of a strange environment. The judicious use of a suitable sedative is beneficial because it provides a stress-free preoperative phase.

Normal thermoregulatory mechanisms are depressed in the elderly. Anaesthetic agents can exacerbate this problem because they decrease the heat-production mechanisms and at the same time increase heat loss (Waterman, 1975; Evans, Sawyer and Krahwinkel, 1973). Hypothermic episodes can develop rapidly in geriatric patients during anaesthesia unless preventative measures are taken (Gravenstein and Paulus, 1982).

Cardiovascular system

Baroreflex activity, blood volume, blood pressure, and cardiac output are decreased in the aged animal. There may also be a physiological vagotonia (Evans, 1981). Older patients are frequently unable to compensate fully for the rapid cardiovascular changes that occur following the administration of intravenous anaesthetic agents and the arm–brain circulation time may be prolonged. It is important that the total dose of these agents be reduced accordingly and that they be administered slowly and to effect. The loss of baroreflex activity results in a diminished response to intraoperative blood loss, and this may potentiate anaesthetic-induced hypotension.

Cardiac degenerative changes are common and are often progressive in older animals. One study demonstrated a 25% incidence of heart disease in dogs between 9 and 12 years old and a 33% incidence in dogs 13 years and older (MacDougall and Barker, 1984). Many of the degenerative cardiac lesions reported are associated with chronic valvular disease (MacDougall and Barker, 1984). Endocardiosis is particularly prevalent in small breeds of dog. The pathology is that of a progressive, degenerative lesion of the heart valves and support apparatus. Valvular regurgitation, especially of the atrioventricular valves, occurs because of the deposition of acid mucopolysaccharides and results in valvular insufficiency. There is an increase in myocardial work and oxygen demand and, in severe cases, there may be myocardial hypoxia (Bonagura, 1981). Heart failure is a long-term sequela to endocardiosis.

Other acquired diseases that may be present in geriatric dogs include cor pulmonale in brachycephalic breeds, sick sinus syndrome in Miniature Schnauzers, and supraventricular dysrhythmias in giant breeds. In aged cats, hypertrophic cardiomyopathy secondary to hyperthyroidism and endocardiosis are probably the most commonly diagnosed forms of cardiovascular disease.

Cardiovascular disease can usually be diagnosed from the clinical history and thorough preoperative examination. Appropriate medical management of clinically significant cardiovascular conditions should be instituted before anaesthesia.

Respiratory system

Pulmonary function deteriorates progressively with increasing age. This decline is secondary to physical changes that occur in both the lungs and chest wall. One of the most significant changes that has been measured in dogs is a decrease in lung elasticity (Robinson and Gillespie, 1973). It can be argued that a loss of elastic recoil will result in an increase in the lung volume at which small airways begin to close (the closing volume). Evans (1981) states that this has been demonstrated in dogs.

In humans at rest in the supine position, the closing volume begins to exceed the functional residual capacity at the age of 45 years (Don, 1971). Changes of this magnitude cause significant ventilation–perfusion disturbances and will tend to produce hypoxaemia by increasing the alveolar to arterial oxygen tension difference. Raine (1965) demonstrated a progressive deterioration of Pao_2 with age in humans, and a similar relationship may apply in animals.

With advancing age in humans, the pulmonary vasculature undergoes fibrosis, bronchial and chondral cartilages calcify, the thoracic wall stiffens, and mechanical ventilatory function and reserves are reduced (Miller, 1981). Evaluation of thoracic radiographs of old dogs often reveals similar anatomical changes, which presumably contribute to reduced ventilatory function. These changes include an increased density of the bronchovascular pattern, intrapleural calcification, and costochondral calcification. The diffusion capacity of the lungs and pulmonary capillary blood volume have been demonstrated to decrease with increasing age in dogs (Robinson and Gillespie, 1975).

Auscultation of the lung fields of older animals and humans (Robertson, 1980) usually reveals an increase in vesicular lung sounds and, sometimes, wheezing. The increased lung sounds are generally attributed to turbulence caused by narrowing of the small airways, although in human studies it has been shown that there is little change in total airway resistance with advancing age (Miller, 1981). The increase in resistance associated with small airway narrowing may be balanced by a decrease in upper airway resistance. In support of this, the diameter of both the larynx and trachea have been reported to increase with age (Evans, 1973). As might be projected, anatomical and physiological dead space both increase with age in humans (Evans, 1973; Miller, 1981) and the same is probably true in animals. Another change that has been shown to occur in elderly people, but has not been demonstrated in animals, is that the protective airway reflexes become less active (Pontoppidan and Beecher, 1960).

The changes discussed above are normal degenerative ageing changes, but they are sometimes complicated by chronic pulmonary disease. Chronic bronchitis is the most common form of chronic pulmonary disease and is the end result of most unresolved pulmonary diseases. The history is one of chronic coughing and excess mucus production. The disease presents mainly in small dog breeds and may be associated with a collapsing trachea (Wheeldon, 1974). Another potential problem in geriatric dogs is pulmonary neoplasia. Tumours of all types are more common in older animals, and malignant tumours frequently metastasize to the lungs. A primary tumour and a history of coughing or weight loss should alert the clinician to this possibility. Other pulmonary diseases are less common but present on occasion. Disease conditions like bronchiectasis, pulmonary fibrosis, emphysema, and allergic bronchitis may be more common in the older dog.

The ageing changes discussed above and any coexisting pulmonary disease will impact adversely on normal gas exchange. This should be borne in mind when anaesthetizing geriatric patients if respiratory complications are to be avoided. Respiratory function of these patients should be improved as far as possible prior to anaesthesia by appropriate medical therapy. When indicated, oxygen enrichment of the inspired air and intermittent positive pressure ventilation are beneficial.

Renal system

Little research has been done on the effects of ageing on the canine kidney, but changes similar to those reported in humans probably occur. These include the following (Ellison, 1975; Miller, 1981; Robertson, 1980):

1. Decreased renal blood flow.
2. Decreased glomerular filtration rate.
3. Reduced ability to concentrate urine.
4. Loss of nephrons.
5. Increased blood urea nitrogen.
6. Renal cortical vascular deterioration with an alteration in distribution of flow from the cortex to the medulla.
7. Impairment of distal tubular function with a reduced ability to handle acid excretion.
8. Increased urinary volume necessary to excrete the obligatory solute load.

Renal function in dogs and cats is often markedly impaired in old age. Older animals frequently are unable to concentrate urine and as a result show signs of polydipsia and polyuria. Gross changes of this nature are often the result of chronic renal disease. Chronic interstitial nephritis and glomerulonephritis feature prominently in the differential diagnosis in dogs (Wright, 1980). In a postmortem survey, it was reported that chronic nephritis, pyelonephritis, and glomerulonephritis accounted for about 5% of canine mortality (Bronson, 1982). Renal disease was the second most common cause of death in this study (cancer was the most common cause of death). In a similar study involving cats, renal disease was implicated in 5% of feline deaths (Bronson, 1981).

Impaired renal function, as a result of old age or intercurrent disease, prolongs the plasma half-life of drugs that are eliminated by the kidney. Anaesthetic agents should be selected with this in mind, particularly if preoperative screening tests indicate renal dysfunction. In addition, close attention should be directed towards maintaining fluid and electrolyte balance in patients with renal dysfunction as the kidney is intimately involved in fluid and electrolyte homeostasis.

Hepatic system

Information regarding age-related changes in liver function is scant and often contradictory. Most of the conventional liver function tests are unchanged in older patients. Plasma sulphobromophthalein sodium (BSP) retention has been shown to increase with age due to selective reduction in the uptake and storage capacity of the liver for BSP (Thompson and Williams, 1965). These changes have been attributed mainly to a reduction in hepatic blood flow (Kitani, 1977). An important corollary of this disturbance is a decrease in plasma clearance of many drugs resulting in prolongation of their pharmacological action.

Fat accumulation in the liver (hepatic lipidosis) is more common in older animals. This change is sometimes secondary to other diseases (e.g. diabetes mellitus, hyperadrenocorticism, and hypothyroidism) and results in hepatomegaly, increases in serum alanine aminotransferase and alkaline phosphatase, and disturbance of liver function (Mosier and Bradley, 1983). Hepatic cirrhosis is also a disease of the older animal because of its chronic and progressive nature. The cause is usually multifactorial, resulting in reduced parenchymal mass and, therefore, functional capacity (Mosier and Bradley, 1983). The liver is sometimes a site of neoplastic disease, with the majority of tumours being primary in origin. Because of the large functional reserve of the normal liver, however, clinical signs are often inapparent until the tumour is widely disseminated (Hardy, 1983). In one study, BSP retention was found to increase by only 6% to 11% in 33% of dogs with hepatocellular carcinomas (Strombeck, 1978).

Endocrine system

Thyroid glands. No significant alterations in the serum levels of triiodothyronine (T_3) or thyroxine (T_4) have been associated with ageing in humans (Olsen, Laurberg and Weeke, 1978). Older dogs, however, appear to have slightly lower serum T_4 levels, although the extent of this change (0.07 mg 100 ml^{-1} a year) may not be clinically significant (Belshaw and Rijnbeck, 1979). Hypothyroidism has been reported to be the most common endocrinopathy in the dog (Rosychuk, 1983). Most cases of canine hypothyroidism are familial and have an early age of onset (two to five years). However, this disease is also common in the older individual (Milne and Hayes, 1981). Hypothyroidism is extremely rare in the cat, except for the iatrogenic form which occurs following surgical or medical thyroid ablation. The important abnormalities that accompany hypothyroidism include (Rosychuk, 1983; Wood, 1983):

1. Thermoregulatory abnormalities (hypothermia).
2. Cardiovascular problems:
   Sinus bradycardia.
   Decreased myocardial contractility.
   Cardiomyopathy.
   Anaemia.
3. Decreased drug metabolism.
4. Obesity.

Hyperthyroidism is a common disorder of middle-aged and older cats but is relatively uncommon in dogs. Pertinent clinical abnormalities associated with this condition include (Peterson, 1987):

1. Cardiovascular disturbances:
   Cardiac murmurs.
   Tachyarrhythmias and premature depolarizations.
   Cardiomyopathy.
2. Temperament changes (hyperexcitability, aggression).
3. Cachexia.

Adrenal glands. Basal or ACTH-stimulated plasma cortisol levels are unchanged with increasing age in humans (Gherondache, Romanoff and Pincus, 1967). Some authors, though, have reported 'adrenal exhaustion' in elderly patients undergoing continued stress, especially during anaesthesia and surgery (Lorhan, 1971; Weidmann *et al.*, 1975). It has been suggested that supplementary corticosteroids be administered to geriatric animals prior to surgery (Evans, 1981). Renin and aldosterone secretion appear to be attenuated in response to stress in geriatric people (Weidmann *et al.*, 1975). The biological significance and pathogenic mechanisms of these changes are unclear (Davis and Davis, 1983). These hormones play a key role in the control of water, sodium, and potassium balance, and blood pressure.

Hyperadrenocorticism is a relatively common endocrine disorder of middle-aged and older dogs (Feldman, 1983). The major problems associated with this condition include muscle weakness, marked reduction in expiratory reserve volume, decreased chest wall compliance, expanded vascular volume (possibly leading to congestive heart failure) and pyelonephritis (Feldman, 1983). Dogs on chemotherapy (*o,p'*-DDD) may also develop iatrogenic mineralocorticoid deficiency, giving rise to severe electrolyte disturbances.

Plasma noradrenaline (norepinephrine) levels increase with age due to a decline in plasma clearance (Martin and Capen, 1979). This would suggest increased cardiovascular instability, but the change is probably balanced by a decrease in noradrenaline receptor sensitivity (Davis and Davis, 1983). Adrenaline levels remain unchanged with age (Esler and Shews, 1981).

Pancreas. Glucose tolerance decreases with age, possibly because of a decline in insulin receptor responsiveness or a reduction in the number of receptors (Davis and Davis, 1983). Diabetes mellitus is most common in older dogs and cats (Feldman and Nelson, 1986; Nelson and Feldman, 1986). The complications associated with this disease include osmotic diuresis, concurrent infectious diseases, liver diesase (fat deposition and cirrhosis) and keto-acidosis (Franco-Morselli *et al.*, 1977).

Hyperinsulinism associated with functional beta cell tumours is most common in older dogs (8 to 12 years of age). Hypoglycaemia may be a problem in these animals during anaesthesia necessitating periodic intraoperative blood glucose assay and intravenous glucose administration if required (Feldman, 1983).

Pituitary gland. Antidiuretic hormone secretion increases with age in humans to compensate for decreased sensitivity of receptors in the distal renal tubules (Helderman *et al.*, 1978). Impaired renal concentrating ability, which has been described in elderly human patients, may be a consequence of the decrease in receptor sensitivity (Davis and Davis, 1983). Similar changes may occur in elderly animals.

ANAESTHETIC MANAGEMENT OF THE GERIATRIC PATIENT

A clinical history should be elicited from the owner and a thorough physical examination should be performed before anaesthesia. Ideally, blood is taken for a complete blood cell count and chemistry profile at this time. In otherwise healthy geriatric patients, haematocrit, total serum protein, serum urea nitrogen (or creatinine), and blood glucose are considered the minimum pre-operative laboratory database.

Local analgesia

Local or regional analgesia, which is normally much safer than general anaesthesia, is highly recommended in extremely old and decrepit patients. Chemical restraint may be required to facilitate patient handling. Intravenous regional analgesia can be employed for procedures involving the distal limbs. This technique is easy to perform and involves the intravenous injection of a local anaesthetic solution distal to a tourniquet. Blood levels of the local anaesthetic following release of the tourniquet are well below those considered to be toxic (Bogan and Weaver, 1978).

Another technique that is relatively simple to perform is epidural analgesia. Local analgesic solution is injected into the epidural space, usually at the level of the lumbosacral junction. Anterior epidural block extending to the midthoracic region is associated with paralysis of sympathetic fibres that give rise to the coeliac and anterior mesenteric ganglia. This results in hypotension which may be severe in the aged animal because the adaptive capacity of the cardiovascular system is limited. Hypotension can be avoided by preloading the patient with 20–30 ml kg^{-1} of a crystalloid solution or by the administration of an α-adrenergic agonist (e.g. methoxamine). Careful monitoring of the pulse and capillary refill time is required throughout the procedure. Rostral spread of local analgesic solution to the level of the first thoracic vertebra should be avoided as it will result in blockade of the cardioaccelerator nerves and prevent the normal cardiovascular response to hypotension. If hypotension does occur, it should be treated with intravenous fluids and/or a vasopressor.

There are several nerve block sites around the head that can be used for oral or facial surgery. Unfortunately, even if analgesia is complete, most dogs will not be cooperative enough to permit surgery.

General anaesthesia

Preoperative preparation. Prior to anaesthesia, dogs and cats should have food withheld for 8 to 12 hours and should be denied access to water for one to two hours. It is particularly important not to deprive older animals of fluid for prolonged periods. Uraemic crisis may develop more rapidly in older patients because of their relatively low blood volume and reduced ability to concentrate urine.

Premedication. Low doses of acepromazine (0.025–0.05 mg kg^{-1} i.m.) are usually satisfactory for sedative premedication of otherwise healthy geriatric animals. Acepromazine produces mild and reliable sedation in the elderly patient and is comparatively safe. It should, however, be avoided in animals with cardiovascular disturbances, such as congestive cardiac failure secondary to valvular endocardiosis or cardiomyopathy. In these patients, the α-adrenoceptor blocking effect of acepromazine may cause a precipitous fall in blood pressure, and possibly syncope. Acepromazine should also be avoided in animals prone to seizures as it may lower the cerebral convulsive threshold.

Butorphanol, a synthetic opioid analgesic, is an alternative agent that can be used for premedication. It can be given intramuscularly at a dose rate of 0.05–0.2 mg kg⁻¹. The sedation it produces is mild but useful. Butorphanol causes little myocardial depression or change in vascular tone. However, in common with other opioids, it has a tendency to produce bradycardia. For this reason, it should be administered with an anticholinergic agent, such as atropine or glycopyrronium (glycopyrrolate). If the resting heart rate is high and atropine-induced tachycardia is considered undesirable, glycopyrronium may be preferable. Respiratory depression, characteristic of opioids, is limited with butorphanol, reaching a plateau of effect at a relatively low dose rate. Should a crisis of any kind occur, butorphanol can be reversed with an opioid antagonist such as naloxone (0.02–0.04 mg kg⁻¹ i.v).

Neuroleptanalgesic combinations, such as fentanyl-droperidol, can be used in low dosages for premedicating fractious dogs. The opioid component may be reversed with naloxone. This is an advantage when dealing with geriatric patients in which the response to a drug or drug combination cannot always be predicted.

Induction. Inhalation induction of anaesthesia with halothane or isoflurane is a safe technique in the geriatric patient. These anaesthetic agents are administered in a controlled manner in an oxygen-enriched atmosphere and, should any complications arise, recovery is rapid following discontinuation of anaesthetic administration. Excitement is a potential problem during inhalation induction, but may be minimized or avoided by gentle handling of the patient, gradual introduction of the anaesthetic agent, and appropriate preanaesthetic sedation.

Halothane is probably the most widely used inhalation induction agent, although isoflurane offers several advantages. The relatively low blood solubility of isoflurane makes anaesthetic induction and recovery extremely rapid. Also, isoflurane does not potentiate the arrhythmogenic effect of adrenaline on the heart, which is valuable at induction when catecholamine levels are often elevated. Isoflurane does, however, have a pungent odour, so that high concentrations may cause some resistance by the animal.

Injectable anaesthetics offer the advantage of allowing rapid induction of anaesthesia and may be titrated to effect when used intravenously. These agents are normally safe if used correctly. However, there are certain provisions which should be borne in mind when using these agents in geriatric patients. Older patients often have reduced cerebral function, slowed circulation, reduced blood volume, decreased hepatorenal function, muscle wasting and reduced body fat. These changes will affect the activity, distribution and elimination of intravenous induction agents, tending to increase their potency and duration of effect.

If thiobarbiturates are used in geriatric patients, they should be administered in smaller increments than normal, possibly starting with a test dose of 1 mg kg^{-1} i.v. to determine the sensitivity of the animal to the drug. To avoid prolonged recovery which may be associated with exclusive thiobarbiturate induction, inhalation anaesthetic agents may be administered to complete induction following a small ('sleep') dose of thiobarbiturate. Methohexitone also may be used to induce anaesthesia in geriatric animals. It is rapidly metabolized and recovery is shorter than with thiobarbiturates, but it can cause profound cardiorespiratory depression if injected too rapidly. On the other hand, slow injection of methohexitone may cause excitement, particularly in inadequately premedicated animals. Premedication with opioids or ataractics will minimize this potential problem.

Opioid analgesics and neuroleptanalgesic mixtures may be used to induce anaesthesia in old or debilitated dogs. Sedative premedication is not mandatory but improves the quality of induction when opioids are used in this way. Oxymorphone is commonly used for this type of induction at a dosage of between 0.1 and 0.3 mg kg^{-1} i.v. (Sawyer, 1982). The quality of induction is fair in most elderly patients.

Respiratory depression at induction is a complication of all the methods described. For geriatric patients, which have increased sensitivity to anaesthetic drugs and reduced pulmonary function, it is best to preoxygenate for two to three minutes prior to induction. This ensures that hypoxaemia does not complicate the induction period.

Intubation. A snug-fitting endotracheal tube should be inserted into the airway and the cuff inflated immediately after induction. It may be possible to use a slightly wider endotracheal tube than anticipated because of the relatively wider laryngeal and tracheal diameter in the elderly patient.

Maintenance. Inhalation maintenance is safest for geriatric patients. Breathing may be spontaneous or controlled. Spontaneous breathing techniques are satisfactory for the majority of older animals, particularly if they are healthy and if the proposed operative procedure is short. In extremely old and debilitated patients undergoing major surgery, it is advisable to control ventilation to ensure that hypoventilation does not occur and to eliminate the work of breathing. Intermittent positive ventilation of the lungs (IPPV) can be performed by manually squeezing the reservoir bag or by means of a mechanical ventilator.

Isoflurane is probably the best inhalation agent currently available for maintenance of anaesthesia for reasons cited previously. It is expensive, however, and a precision vaporizer for isoflurane requires considerable capital outlay. For those experienced in its use, halothane can provide safe anaesthesia for physiologically compromised patients. The inspired halothane concentration is reduced by up to 22% in the dog if 60–70% nitrous oxide is used in the background gas mixture (DeYoung and Sawyer, 1980). Care must be taken to ensure adequate oxygenation of the patient if nitrous oxide is used. There should always be at least 30% oxygen in the inspired gas mixture. This is particularly important in geriatric patients because of their reduced pulmonary function.

If ventilation is controlled, it is a relatively simple matter to give a neuromuscular blocking agent intravenously should supplementary muscle relaxation or reflex movement suppression be required. This is more acceptable than increasing the depth of anaesthesia in a debilitated patient. This type of anaesthesia involving the use of IPPV and muscle relaxants is known as balanced anaesthesia. Physiological depression is minimized because only low levels of potent inhalation agents are used. Balanced anaesthesia requires close supervision by a trained person.

Supportive therapy. Intravenous fluids should be administered to geriatric patients throughout anaesthesia in quantities sufficient to maintain blood volume and urine flow. An infusion rate of approximately 10 ml kg^{-1} h^{-1} is sufficient for most procedures and rarely causes any problems. This rate of infusion may be excessive in the presence of heart failure or anuric renal failure. A simple way of ensuring the appropriate infusion rate is to monitor the central venous pressure. Urinary output can also be a guide and should be maintained at greater than 0.3 ml kg^{-1} h^{-1} (Osborne, Low and Sinco, 1972).

A heating pad or circulating warm water blanket should be positioned under the patient soon after the induction of anaesthesia to prevent hypothermia. Animals at either extreme of age, especially small breeds of dog and cats, are susceptible to hypothermia (Waterman, 1975). Recovery from anaesthesia may be considerably prolonged if the body temperature falls by even a few degrees.

Monitoring. It is important to monitor the following parameters at frequent intervals throughout anaesthesia:

1. Heart rate and rhythm (by oesophageal stethoscope).
2. Respiratory rate and character.

3. Pulse rate and quality.
4. Colour of mucous membranes.
5. Capillary refill time.
6. Electrocardiogram.
7. Rectal temperature.

In some cases it is also valuable to monitor arterial pressure (indirect or direct), urinary output, haematocrit, total serum protein and blood gases.

Recovery. Recovery should be supervised in all patients. Supervision is particularly important in geriatric patients because they tolerate physiological insults poorly. Geriatric patients should receive oxygen supplementation and fluid therapy until they have fully recovered consciousness. Humane measures, such as the provision of analgesia and a comfortable environment, are also important to minimize stress and help to ensure a pleasant as well as an uneventful recovery.

REFERENCES

Belshaw, B. E. and Rijnbeck, A. (1979). *Journal of the American Animal Hospital Association* **15**, 17.

Bogan, J. A. and Weaver, A. D. (1978). *American Journal of Veterinary Research* **39**, 1672.

Bonagura, J. D. (1981). *Veterinary Clinics of North America* **11**, 705.

Bronson, R. T. (1981). *American Journal of Veterinary Research* **42**, 1606.

Bronson, R. T. (1982). *American Journal of Veterinary Research* **43**, 2057.

Davis, P. J. and Davis, F. B. (1983). In *Clinical Aspects of Aging*, ed. W. Reichel, pp. 396–410. Baltimore: The Williams & Wilkins Co.

DeYoung, D. J. and Sawyer, D. C. (1980). *Journal of the American Animal Hospital Association* **16**, 125.

Don, H. (1971). *Anesthesiology* **35**, 582.

Eger, E. I. (1974). *Anesthesia Uptake and Action.* Baltimore: The Williams & Wilkins Co.

Ellison, N. (1975). *Surgical Clinics of North America* **55**, 929.

Esler, M. and Shews, H. (1981). *Clinical Science* **60**, 217.

Evans, T. I. (1973). *Anaesthesia and Intensive Care* **1**, 319.

Evans, T. (1981). *Veterinary Clinics of North America* **11**, 653.

Evans, A. T., Sawyer, D. C. and Krahwinkel, D. J. (1973). *Journal of the American Veterinary Medical Association* **163**, 147.

Feldman, E. C. (1983). In *Textbook of Veterinary Internal Medicine*,

Diseases of the Dog and Cat, ed. S. J. Ettinger, pp. 1650–1696. Philadelphia: W. B. Saunders Co.

Feldman, E. C. and Nelson, R. W. (1986). In *Current Veterinary Therapy IX. Small Animal Practice*, ed. R. W. Kirk, p. 1000. Philadelphia: W. B. Saunders Co.

Franco-Morselli, R., Elghozi J. L., Joly, E., Di Giuilio, S. and Myer, P. (1977). *British Medical Journal* **ii**, 1251.

Gherondache, C. N., Romanoff, L. P. and Pincus, G. (1967). In *Endocrines and Aging*, ed. L. Gitman, p. 76. Springfield, IL: Charles C. Thomas.

Gravenstein, J. S. and Paulus, D. A. (1982). *Monitoring Practice in Clinical Anesthesia*, p. 166. Philadelphia: J. B. Lippincott Co.

Hardy, R. M. (1983). In *Textbook of Veterinary Internal Medicine*, ed. S. J. Ettinger, pp. 1372–1434. Philadelphia: W. B. Saunders Co.

Helderman, J. H., Vestal, R. E., Rowe, J. W., Tobin, J. D., Andres, R. and Robertson, G. L. (1978). *Journal of Gerontology* **33**, 39.

Janis, K. M. (1979). *American Society of Anesthesiologists Refresh Courses* **7**, 143.

Kitani, K. (1977). In *Liver and Aging: Fourth International Giessener Symposium on Experimental Gerontology*, ed D. Platt, pp. 5–17.

Lorhan, P. H. (1971). In *Anesthesia for the Aged*, ed. P. H. Lorhan, pp. 31–33. Springfield IL: Charles C. Thomas.

MacDougall, D. F. and Barker, J. (1984). *British Veterinary Journal* **140**, 115.

Martin, S. I. and Capen, C. C. (1979). In *Canine Medicine*, ed. E. J. Catcott, pp. 1087–1205. Santa Barbara: American Veterinary Publications.

Miller, R. D. (1981). In *Anesthesia*, ed. R. D. Miller, pp. 1231–1246. New York: Churchill Livingstone.

Milne, K. L. and Hayes, H. M. Jr (1981). *Cornell Veterinarian* **71**, 3.

Mosier, J. E. and Bradley, W. D. (1983). In *Textbook of Veterinary Internal Medicine*, ed. S. J. Ettinger, pp. 1372–1434. Philadelphia: W. B. Saunders Co.

Muravchick, S. and Mandel, J. (1982). *Anesthesiology* (Suppl) **57**, A327.

Nelson, R. W. and Feldman, E. C. (1986). In *Current Veterinary Therapy IX. Small Animal Practice*, ed. R. W. Kirk, p. 991. Philadelphia: W. B. Saunders Co.

Olsen, T., Laurberg, P. and Weeke, J. (1978). *Journal of Clinical Endocrinology and Metabolism* **47**, 1111.

Osborne, C. A., Low, D. G. and Sinco, D. R. (1972). *Canine and Feline Urology*, p. 41. Philadelphia: W. B. Saunders Co.

Owens, W. D. (1983). *American Society of Anesthesiologists, 34th Annual Refresher Course Lectures and Clinical Update Program*, p. 228.

Peterson, M. E. (1987). In *Principles and Practice of Veterinary*

Anesthesia, ed. C. E. Short, p. 251. Philadelphia: W. B. Saunders Co.

Pontoppidan, H. and Beecher, H. K. (1960). *Journal of the American Medical Association* **174**, 2209.

Raine, J. M. (1965). *Medical Journal of Australia* **1**, 791.

Roberston, J. D. (1980). In *General Anaesthesia*, 4th edn, eds. T. C. Gray, J. F. Nunn, J. E. Utting, pp. 1453–1473. London: Butterworths.

Robinson, N. E. and Gillespie, J. R. (1973). *Journal of Applied Physiology* **35**, 317.

Robinson, N. E. and Gillespie, J. R. (1975). *Journal of Applied Physiology* **38**, 647.

Rosychuk, R. (1983). In *Current Therapy VIII*, ed. R. W. Kirk, pp. 869–876. Philadelphia: W. B. Saunders Co.

Sawyer, D. C. (1982). *The Practice of Small Animal Anesthesia*, p. 20. Philadelphia: W. B. Saunders Co.

Strombeck, D. R. (1978). *Journal of the American Veterinary Medical Association* **173**, 267.

Swallow, J. J. (1973). MVM thesis, Glasgow University.

Thompson, E. and Williams, R. (1965). *Gut* **6**, 266.

Waterman, A. E. (1975). *Veterinary Record* **96**, 308.

Weidmann, P., De Myttenaere-Bursztein, S., Maxwell, M. H. and de Lima, J. (1975). *Kidney International* **8**, 325.

Wheeldon, E. B. (1974). *Veterinary Record* **94**, 466.

Wood, G. C. (1983). In *Current Veterinary Therapy VIII*, ed. R. W. Kirk, p. 328. Philadelphia: W. B. Saunders Co.

Wright, N. G. (1980). Personal communications, Glasgow University.

3

Anaesthesia for the traumatized patient

Traumatized animals comprise up to 10% of the caseload in some small animal hospitals (Kolata, Kraut and Johnson, 1973). According to one survey, the most common injuries in dogs and cats are those to the head (32–47%), the pelvis (13%), the thorax (11%) and abdomen (9%) (Kolata, 1981). The incidence of airway and pulmonary trauma was reported to be 30% in patients requiring orthopaedic treatment (Tamas *et al.*, 1983). Of these, 40–50% had pulmonary contusion, 15% had pneumothorax and 10% had pleural effusion. Approximately 5% of dogs and cats die as a result of their injuries (Kolata, 1981). Haemorrhage, respiratory insufficiency and injury to the central nervous system (CNS) have been implicated as factors commonly contributing to death (Kolata, 1981). One study found that over 50% of dogs destroyed as a result of trauma had CNS injury (Kolata and Johnson, 1975).

In this chapter, the pathophysiological effects of trauma on the respiratory, cardiovascular and central nervous systems will be reviewed, and the implications of these disturbances for the anaesthetic management of the patient discussed. Special considerations will also be described for specific injuries.

PREANAESTHETIC CONSIDERATIONS

Regardless of the apparent severity of lesions, each patient should undergo rapid assessment of respiratory, cardiovascular and central nervous system function. This will identify imminently life-threatening problems and allow adequate stabilization of the patient before anaesthesia.

Respiratory system

Respiratory dysfunction following trauma commonly results from pulmonary contusion, pneumothorax and pleural effusions. Other

Table 1.   Normal ranges of respiratory parameters

Parameter	Range of values Dog	Cat
Rate (breaths min⁻¹)	10–30	24–42
Tidal volume (ml kg⁻¹)	10–20	10–20
Minute volume (ml kg⁻¹ min⁻¹)	170–350	200–350
Arterial Po_2(mmHg)	85–105	100–115
Arterial Pco_2(mmHg)	30–44	28–35
Arterial pH	7.36–7.46	7.34–7.43
Base deficit (mEq l⁻¹)	0 to −4	−1 to −8

causes of post-traumatic respiratory insufficiency include airway obstruction, chest wall injuries, diaphragmatic hernia and pulmonary oedema. Pulmonary oedema may result from direct lung injury or from CNS injury (Haskins, 1984). The primary mechanism of neurogenic pulmonary oedema is unknown, but may be associated with increased sympathetic activity, which causes a sudden redistribution of blood into the pulmonary circulation (Shapiro, 1986b).

Traumatic injury to the respiratory system frequently results in hypoxaemia and respiratory acidosis although pain, anxiety and the action of vasoactive peptides on pulmonary J-receptors may induce respiratory alkalosis in some patients (Freeman and Nunn, 1963; Douglas *et al.*, 1976). Hypoxaemia results from diffusion abnormalities, shunt and ventilation/perfusion mismatching. Hypercapnia results from hypoventilation and ventilation/perfusion disturbances. Wilson *et al.* (1970) report that ventilation/perfusion mismatching is the most common pulmonary dysfunction associated with trauma in man.

Preliminary assessment of the airway and ventilatory status is based on evaluation of the colour of the mucous membranes, auscultation of the chest and observation of the rate, depth and character of ventilation. Normal respiratory parameters for dogs and cats are given in Table 1. Ventilatory function can be difficult to assess clinically and blood gas analysis may be needed to make a definitive determination.

Where emergency treatment for ventilatory failure is required, a patent airway should be established by endotracheal intubation or tracheostomy. Alveolar ventilation should be assisted by intermittent positive pressure ventilation (IPPV) using an Ambu bag or an anaesthetic circuit. The chest wall should be stabilized and open thoracic wall wounds sealed with petrolatum soaked dressings, sutures or towel clamps. When there is a pneumothorax or haemothorax, lung expansion may be improved by aspiration of

Table 2. Normal ranges of cardiovascular parameters

	Range of values	
Parameter	Dog	Cat
ECG rhythm	Sinus	Sinus
Heart rate (beats min⁻¹)	70–140	110–140
Mean arterial blood pressure	90–110	110–150
Central venous pressure (cmH₂O)	0–10	0–10
Mucous membrane colour	Pink	Pink
Capillary refill time (s)	<2	<2
Core temperature (°C)	37–40	37–40
Core–skin temp. gradient (°C)	<6	<6
(°F)	<10	<10
Urinary output (ml kg⁻¹ h⁻¹)	1–2	1–2

free air or fluid from the pleural space by a tube thoracostomy and suctioning, or by direct needle aspiration (Berkwitt and Berzon, 1985). Oxygenation can be supplemented by conventional means (Court, Dodman and Seeler, 1985.) Following preliminary assessment and initial resuscitation, thoracic radiography should be performed to determine the success of therapy and define abnormalities.

Cardiovascular system

Traumatized patients frequently present with signs of peripheral circulatory failure. Traumatic shock results from a combination of haemorrhage, plasma loss into damaged tissues and pain-mediated inhibition of the vasomotor centre which reduces peripheral vascular tone and venous return (Guyton, 1986). Mean arterial pressure (MAP) and cardiac output (CO) are maintained until a 10% volume deficit is incurred (Guyton, 1986). When a 10–20% volume deficit is incurred, arterioles and venules constrict so that MAP is maintained, but CO decreases (Guyton, 1986). Blood is diverted from 'non-essential' areas to those which are necessary for immediate, short-term survival. Cerebral and myocardial blood flow are preserved at the expense of splanchnic, renal and cutaneous perfusion. Sustained ischaemia of tissue leads to the development of metabolic acidosis and, eventually, irreversible cellular damage.

The patients' circulatory status should be assessed clinically and measures should be taken to restore abnormal values to within the acceptable physiological range. Normal ranges for various cardiovascular parameters in the dog and cat are listed in Table 2.

Rapid administration of intravenous fluids is the mainstay of therapy in traumatic shock. The fluid type is chosen according to the extent of the deficit in circulating fluid volume. Crystalloid solutions, such as lactated Ringer's solution, are used for volume replacement when deficits are mild to moderate and the dose should be approximately three times that of the estimated blood loss (Pascoe, 1987). Moderate signs of shock become apparent when 20–30% of the blood volume is lost and dogs presented in moderate to severe shock require an initial loading dose of crystal-loids of 90 ml kg^{-1} (Pascoe, 1987). For cats in a similar condition, an initial dose of 60 ml kg^{-1} has been recommended (Pascoe, 1987). Crystalloids remain in the intravascular space for approximately 20 minutes before diffusing to the extravascular space. Additional fluid therapy should follow the initial bolus dose to achieve or maintain the circulating blood volume.

Rapid infusion of large volumes of crystalloids will cause significant haemodilution. When the serum total solids concentration falls below 3.5 g dl^{-1}, colloid solutions such as dextrans or plasma should be administered to maintain the intravascular volume and colloid osmotic pressure (Haskins, 1987). High molecular weight dextrans, such as dextran 75, osmotically attract fluid from the extravascular compartment into the intravascular space. The associated blood volume expansion generally exceeds the volume of fluids administered. Dextran 75 should be given at doses of up to but not exceeding 20 ml kg^{-1} within a 24-hour period (Raffe, 1987).

Blood transfusions are indicated when the haematocrit falls acutely below 20% or when 20% or more of the blood volume has been lost (Haskins, 1987; Raffe, 1987). Transfusions of cross-matched fresh whole blood are required in order to maintain adequate oxygen-carrying capacity and provide replacement clotting factors. Fresh whole blood is administered at a dose of up to 40–60 ml kg^{-1} or until the oxygen-carrying capacity of the blood is optimized (Clark, 1982). This is thought to occur when the haematocrit is approximately 30% (Savino and Del Guercio, 1985). When used as a component of shock therapy, blood should be administered in conjunction with a balanced electrolyte solution in a ratio of 1 volume of blood with between 2 and 6 volumes of electrolyte solution (Clark, 1982).

The rate of fluid replacement should be as rapid as the patient will tolerate. Maximal fluid administration rates of 70 ml kg^{-1} h^{-1} have been suggested (Pascoe, 1987). Rapid flows are best achieved using wide-bore, short intravenous catheters with tapered tips (Hoelzer, 1986). More than one intravenous catheter may be needed to achieve rapid fluid administration rates and to allow several types of infusion to be run simultaneously. Preoperative placement of catheters is important since it is difficult to place catheters intraoperatively in an emergency situation when catheterization sites may be inaccessible.

Supplemental use of cardiovascular support agents may be lifesaving when the circulation is failing in spite of fluid therapy. Dopamine or dobutamine are inotropic agents which can be used for circulatory support. An infusion rate of 2–10 μg kg^{-1} min^{-1} of either agent should enhance CO. Dopamine can also be used at low infusion rates (1–2 μg kg^{-1} min^{-1}) to increase blood flow to the renal and splanchnic circulation. The infusion rate of these agents is critical and a balance should be maintained between beneficial effects and deleterious effects of increased cardiac work and oxygen consumption. Other agents suggested for use in shock therapy include corticosteroids, α-adrenoceptor antagonists, fructose and opioid antagonists. The use of corticosteroids is controversial. They are credited with increasing CO, reducing vasoconstriction, stabilizing cell membranes, reducing lactate production and shifting the oxygen–haemoglobin dissociation curve so that oxygen release to peripheral tissues is improved (Massion, 1974). Dexamethasone at doses of 2–6 mg kg^{-1} i.v. over 2–3 minutes or prednisolone sodium succinate at doses of 30–60 mg kg^{-1} i.v. over 2–3 minutes every 8 hours have been recommended (Pascoe, 1987). α-Adrenoreceptor antagonists may improve capillary flow, overcome peripheral sludging, and increase venous return, providing fluid deficits have been corrected. Phenoxybenzamine and phentolamine have been successfully used in patients with severe shock and intense vasoconstriction (Clark, 1982). Fructose-1,6-diphosphate improves haemodynamic and pulmonary function, possibly by enhancing anaerobic carbohydrate metabolism and reducing tissue injury from toxic oxygen radicals generated by neutrophils (Markoo, 1986). Opioid antagonists may also improve cardiovascular function in hypovolaemic patients although high doses are required (McIntosh and Faden, 1986).

Central nervous system

Probably the most common and concerning sequela of head injury for the anaesthetist is increased intracranial pressure (ICP). This may result from intracranial haemorrhage or cerebral oedema. There are no pathognomonic signs for increased ICP but, in man, frequently associated symptoms and signs include headache, nausea, papilloedema, unilateral pupillary dilatation and oculomotor and abducens palsy (Shapiro, 1986a). Changes in the level of consciousness and irregular respiratory patterns denote marked elevations in ICP. Elevation of ICP perpetuates and exacerbates neuronal damage by inducing neural ischaemia, anoxia and oedema. Head trauma may also have detrimental effects on the respiratory and cardiovascular systems. Depending on the site and severity of the lesion, direct trauma to the brain stem may cause any one of a number of respiratory abnormalities including Cheyne–Stokes respiration, hyperventilation, hypoventilation or irregular respiratory patterns. Studies in man indicate a 25% incidence of hypoxaemia associated with head trauma (Shapiro, 1986a). Aetiological factors involved in the development of hypoxaemia include aspiration pneumonia, iatrogenic fluid overload, acute respiratory distress syndrome and neurogenic pulmonary oedema. Hypoventilation causes hypercapnia. This, in turn, increases cerebral blood flow by causing intracranial vasodilatation and results in a further elevation in ICP.

Other sequelae of head trauma which have been reported in man include disseminated intravascular coagulation, pituitary disorders, non-ketotic hyperglycaemia and gastrointestinal haemorrhage (Shapiro, 1986a). Electrocardiographic abnormalities associated with autonomic imbalance also have been observed following head trauma in human patients (Shapiro, 1986a). These include tachydsyrhythmias and severe atropine-responsive bradycardias. Systemic hypertension may result from excessive sympathetic discharge.

Spinal injuries are associated with physiological sequelae which may pose serious anaesthetic problems. Respiratory disturbances and failure has been reported as a major cause of morbidity and mortality in human patients with acute spinal injury (Smith, 1987). The degree of respiratory impairment is related to the site of injury and is greatest when the cervical cord is damaged. The diaphragm, which generates the majority of the inspiratory force, is innervated by the phrenic nerve. This nerve is formed by the union of the fifth, sixth and seventh cervical nerves in dogs and damage to these nerves may result in ventilatory failure. Injury to the lower cervical cord and upper thorcic cord may remove abdominal and intercostal ventilatory support, reduce the expiratory reserve capacity and leave the patient with little or no ability to cough. These patients usually develop hypoxaemia or atelectasis secondary to hypoventilation or pneumonia. Gastric dilatation caused by autonomic dysfunction associated with spinal injury and aspiration may impair ventilatory function further in patients with spinal cord damage.

Spinal injury may induce cardiovascular derangements. Preganglionic sympathetic nerves exit the spinal cord of the dog as far caudally as the fifth lumbar segment. Spinal cord injury above this segment may interrupt sympathetic outflow to the peripheral vasculature causing hypotension. In addition, injury to the upper thoracic cord may interrupt the sympathetic flow to the heart, resulting in bradycardia and reduced haemodynamic reserve. The limited haemodynamic reserve of these patients makes them extremely sensitive to volume changes and susceptible to pulmonary oedema.

Elevations in serum concentrations of potassium and calcium are common findings in humans with acute spinal cord injury and these electrolyte disturbances have serious implications for cardiac function and anaesthetic management (Smith, 1987).

Spinal shock sometimes occurs as a reaction to spinal trauma. In this syndrome, spinal cord damage interrupts the path of facilitatory impulses from higher centres to neurons below the site of the injury. Without tonic input, the activity of neurons below the site of injury is temporarily subdued and hypotension, bradycardia and delayed gastric emptying are among the possible sequelae. The condition usually resolves within a few to 24 hours when the spinal neurons below the site of damage increase their own excitability and begin functioning again (Guyton, 1986). Loss of thermoregulatory ability is another sequela of spinal injury. Sympathetic nerves carry neurons of the thermo-regulatory pathway from the brain. Disruption of these pathways causes a loss of thermoregulation in those areas of the body supplied by nerves below the site of the lesion and maintenance of body heat may be compromised.

The principles of management of patients with neurological damage are to prevent secondary damage to intact nervous tissue and to support vital functions under the physiological control of damaged tissue. Therapy to minimize nervous tissue damage is directed towards reducing intracranial volume (in the case of head trauma) and neural oedema, and eliminating hypoxaemia. Preoperatively, oxygenation, hyperventilation and mannitol therapy should be instituted when neural damage is suspected (Archibald, Holt and Sokolovsky, 1981). Oxygen supplementation optimizes oxygen delivery to the damaged nervous tissue. Hyperventilation lowers the arterial carbon dioxide tension ($Paco_2$), removing a potent stimulus for cerebral vasodilatation. This reduces intracranial volume and may restore cerebral autoregulation (Henning, 1986). Hyperventilation to a $Paco_2$ of 25–35 mmHg (3.3–4.7 kPa) is adequate in most cases (Bedford and Durbin, 1986). Mannitol reduces neural oedema by an osmotic effect. It should be given slowly intravenously over at least 1 hour at a dose of 1.0–2.0 g kg^{-1} (Archibald *et al.*, 1981). Mannitol should only be used after the blood volume has been replenished in order to avoid dehydration and hypotension which would otherwise result from its diuretic effects. If the blood–brain barrier is incomplete, as may be the case in severe head trauma, mannitol may increase the ICP by leaking into neural tissue.

Other adverse effects of mannitol administration include

vomiting, polydypsia, hyponatraemia, pulmonary oedema, and congestive heart failure (Davis, 1984).

Other considerations

In the majority of cases, once the patient has undergone cardiopulmonary and neurological stabilization, there is time to obtain a more detailed history and to perform a more comprehensive physical assessment. Previous and current illnesses, allergies and previous anaesthetic experiences should be noted.

ANAESTHESIA

The nature and extent of trauma influence the selection of anaesthetic agents and techniques. The following sections will discuss general considerations involved in the formulation of an appropriate anaesthetic regimen for the traumatized small animal patient.

Anaesthetic drug disposition

The pharmacokinetics and pharmacodynamics of anaesthetic agents may be altered by trauma. For example, delayed onset of action of injectable anaesthetic agents should be anticipated in hypovolaemia because of prolonged circulation time and reduced peripheral perfusion. Subcutaneous administration of injectable anaesthetic agents is often unreliable and the intramuscular route should be used in preference, allowing sufficient time for the drug to achieve its maximal effect. In shock, rapid rates of intravenous injection of even small doses of certain anaesthetic drugs may cause severe circulatory depression and these agents are best administered slowly in small incremental doses and to effect (Graves, 1974). The brain and myocardium receive a greater portion of the cardiac output during hypovolaemic states and drug dosages often need to be reduced if relative overdose is to be avoided (Graves, 1974). Decreased splanchnic flow reduces redistribution, metabolism and excretion of many anaesthetic agents and recovery time from anaesthesia may be prolonged (Graves, 1974). In addition, microsomal enzyme activity is often reduced by acute ischaemia, physical injury or burns and the metabolism of anaesthetic agents may be delayed (Kirkwood *et al.*, 1986).

For inhalational agents, the combination of hyperventilation and reduced CO characteristic of traumatic shock permits the alveolar concentration of highly soluble agents such as methoxyflurane to reach high levels rapidly, further depressing the circulation (Eger, 1974). The uptake and distribution of the less soluble agents such as nitrous oxide and isoflurane may be more predictable in low cardiac output states. Patient sensitivity to inhalational anaesthetic agents is increased in hypovolaemic patients. In one study, the halothane minimum alveolar concentration for dogs was shown to be reduced by 20% following a haemorrhagic episode which reduced the MAP by one-third to one-half of control values (Eger, Saidman and Brandstater, 1965).

Premedication

The purposes of premedication are to produce a cooperative patient at induction and to reduce the dose requirement of induction and maintenance agents. For trauma patients, it is also often important to provide adequate analgesia. Excessive doses of premedicants should be avoided because of associated cardiopulmonary depression. Animals in severe shock or those which have respiratory insufficiency may be experiencing a degree of cerebral hypoxia and may appear anxious. In these cases, oxygen supplementation alone will sometimes reduce anxiety and further sedation may be unnecessary.

Opioid agents provide analgesia and some degree of sedation with minimal cardiovascular depression and are useful in traumatized patients despite their mild respiratory depressant effects (Haskins, 1987). Specific antagonist agents should be available in case of complications. Morphine (0.5–1.0 mg kg^{-1} i.m.), pethidine (3.0–5.0 mg kg^{-1} i.m.), oxymorphone (0.05–0.1 mg kg^{-1} i.m.) or butorphanol (0.1–0.4 mg kg^{-1} i.m.) may be used. Use of an anticholinergic agent in conjunction with opioid agents will help to prevent opioid-induced bradycardia.

Low doses of α-adrenoceptor antagonists such as acepromazine and droperidol may be employed as sedatives in traumatized patients providing the blood volume of the patient has been repleted. The antidysrhythmic properties of acepromazine are beneficial when dysrhythmias are present or anticipated.

Ketamine may be used as a premedicant in cats except where neurological or urinary system damage has been sustained. A more detailed description of the advantages and disadvantages of ketamine in trauma patients is provided later in this chapter.

The authors prefer to avoid the use of xylazine in traumatized patients because of its profound respiratory and circulatory depressant effects (Kolata and Rawlings, 1982).

Induction

Volatile anaesthetic agents are relatively safe for induction of general anaesthesia in traumatized, hypovolaemic patients since these agents can be titrated to effect permitting a relatively rapid response to changing haemodynamic circumstances (Clarke and Carson, 1980). Of the available agents, isoflurane causes the least reduction in CO and has the added advantage of not sensitizing the heart to the dysrhythmic action of adrenaline (Hickey and Eger, 1986). Disadvantages of inhalation induction techniques include excitement and stress at induction and increased risk of vomition with aspiration.

In patients with respiratory insufficiency and limited respiratory reserve, it is important to avoid excitement or struggling which may result in hypoxaemia and catecholamine release. Under these circumstances, intravenous induction techniques are preferable to inhalational techniques. Barbiturates are suitable induction agents for haemodynamically stable patients but in hypovolaemic patients these agents have been described as 'ideal agents for euthanasia' (Halford, 1943). Barbiturates are probably best avoided in shock because of their low safety margin. Where cardiovascular stability is a concern in canine patients, the induction of narcosis with an opioid agent should be considered. Preoxygenation is essential when using opioid induction techniques to prevent hypoxaemia. Haskins (1987) has described the use of oxymorphone (0.2–0.6 mg kg^{-1} i.v.) or fentanyl (0.2 mg kg^{-1} i.v.) as induction agents. Either agent is administered in quarter dose increments until the desired effect is achieved. The administration of diazepam (0.2 mg kg^{-1} i.v.) immediately following the first increment of the opioid agent will improve muscle relaxation and suppress hypersensitivity of the patient to noise. Once induction is complete, the patient should be intubated and inspired gases supplemented with oxygen.

Ketamine may be used to induce anaesthesia in traumatized cats providing renal or neurological injury is not present. It has minimal respiratory depressant effects and its sympathomimetic properties enhance CO, MAP, and heart rate in normovolaemic patients (Chasapakis *et al.*, 1973; Bond and Davis, 1974; Lanning and Harmel, 1975; Booth, 1982; Seyde and Longnecker, 1984). The beneficial cardiovascular effects of ketamine depend on the level of pre-existing sympathetic tone. When sympathetic tone is maximal, the direct myocardial depressant effects of ketamine predominate (Traber, Wilson and Priano, 1968). In one study in which animals were depleted of 30% of their blood volume, the best cardiovascular protection was provided by isoflurane; enflurane and halothane were intermediate in terms of cardiovascular stability and the least protection was afforded by ketamine (Priano, 1985). In another study in animals which had between 10 and 30% depletion of blood volume, ketamine produced a greater mismatch between whole body oxygen supply and demand than inhalational agents (Weiskopf, Townsley and Riordan, 1981). Ketamine may not be as safe is it is sometimes perceived to be and should be used cautiously in hypovolaemic patients.

In normal cats, alphaxalone and alphadolone acetate (Saffan, Glaxo, Middlesex) has a high therapeutic index but produces cardiovascular effects similar to those of the barbiturates (Child *et al.*, 1971). Histaminoid reactions associated with the use of Saffan in cats make the agent potentially dangerous in hypovolaemic patients (Child *et al.*, 1971; Corbett, 1976; Dodman, 1980).

Maintenance

Inhalational agents are commonly used for maintenance of anaesthesia in traumatized patients (Clarke and Carson, 1980). For maximal patient support, inhalational anaesthetic agents may be supplemented by nitrous oxide and muscle relaxants in a balanced anaesthetic regimen (Dodman, Seeler and Court, 1984). Nitrous oxide provides analgesia and reduces the requirement for other inhalational gases (Booth, 1982). Unfortunately, the use of this agent reduces the inspired fraction of oxygen and it should be employed cautiously when arterial oxygenation is marginal. Nitrous oxide is contraindicated where closed gas pockets exist, for example, in animals with pneumothorax (Booth, 1982). Incorporation of muscle relaxants into an anaesthetic regimen permits a reduction in the dose of inspired anaesthetic agents (Adams, 1982). The non-depolarizing agents atracurium and vecuronium have little or no adverse effect on the cardiovascular system and should be well tolerated by patients in shock (Miller, 1986; Savarese, 1986).

Opioid agents can be used to maintain anaesthesia in trauma patients by administering small aliquots (oxymorphone, 0.1 mg kg^{-1} i.v.; fentanyl, 0.01 mg kg^{-1} i.v.) every 20 minutes or as required (Haskins, 1987). Diazepam (0.2 mg kg^{-1} i.v.) or a low concentration of an inhalational agent may be administered simultaneously to provide muscle relaxation (Haskins, 1987).

Positioning of the patient is critical in patients with reduced pulmonary function. When the pulmonary lesion is unilateral, the non-functional lung should be placed uppermost to optimize ventilation/perfusion matching (Fishman, 1981). There are two exceptions. One is when the lesion is a consolidated mass, which, if placed uppermost, would compress the lower lobe and decrease the functional lung volume. The other is when the damaged lung contains a fluid which, if placed uppermost, would drain into and compromise the function of the lower lung.

Monitoring

Monitoring the traumatized patient should commence preoperatively and continue into the recovery period. The intensity and type of monitoring will depend on the condition of the patient but most parameters should be recorded every 5 minutes and trends noted (Dodman *et al.*, 1984). Routine monitoring of the ventilatory status may be augmented by periodic measurement of tidal volume or minute volume using a respirometer and by arterial blood gas analysis. Central venous pressure (CVP) and urinary output may be used to supplement routine cardiovascular monitoring techniques. Intraoperative blood loss should be noted and fluid administration adjusted accordingly. Measurement of core body temperature, peripheral temperature and determination of the core-to-periphery temperature gradient are useful indicators of the adequacy of peripheral perfusion.

Supportive therapy

Fluids are administered according to the needs of the patient. Normovolaemic animals require crystalloid infusions at a rate of 5–10 ml kg^{-1} h^{-1}. For hypovolaemic patients, fluids should be administered more rapidly to maintain arterial pressure within the normal range. Excessive haemodilution can be avoided by serial monitoring of the haematocrit and plasma protein concentration.

It is important to maintain normal body temperature in traumatized patients. Heat loss may be greater than normal since large areas of tissue may be exposed and large volumes of fluids are often infused. Intravenous fluids should be warmed and heat loss minimized by the use of warm water blankets, hot water bottles or radiant heat lamps (Haskins, 1981).

Intermittent positive pressure ventilation is an integral part of maximal support techniques. Although IPPV is normally beneficial, adverse effects may occur if the technique is not correctly employed. The use of peak inspiratory pressures of greater than 30 cmH$_2$O may cause a significant decrease in the CO when the chest is closed. Additionally, IPPV may aggravate previously existing barotrauma especially when fragile alveoli or bullae are present (Haskins, 1984). Intermittent positive pressure ventilation should be curtailed or at least the peak inspiratory pressures should be minimized in some patients with pulmonary trauma. Acute re-expansion of chronically collapsed lungs should be avoided since pulmonary oedema has resulted from re-expansion of lungs which have been collapsed for more than several hours (Mahafan, Simon and Huber, 1979; Garson, Dodman and Baker,

1980; Kernodle, DiRaimondo and Fulkerson, 1984; Ray et al., 1984; Marshall, 1986).

Recovery

Patients should be monitored as intensively as possible until physiological parameters have returned to normal. The orotracheal tube should be maintained for as long as possible and the patient should be closely supervised at the time of extubation. Occasionally, sedation and reintubation or a tracheostomy is necessary in patients that are unable to maintain a patent airway when extubated or when continued ventilatory support is required. Oxygen supplementation, fluid therapy and heat should be provided especially in patients with limited respiratory and cardiovascular reserve. Following a thoracotomy, patients require frequent pleural aspiration of air and blood to avoid complications of pneumothorax and haemothorax (Garson et al., 1980).

Provision of postoperative analgesia reduces patient discomfort and may improve pulmonary function when pain limits ventilatory excursions (Spence, 1980). Systemic administration of an opioid agent is sometimes beneficial. Epidural administration of morphine is an alternative technique (Bonath and Saleh, 1985; Heath et al., 1985). For thoracotomies in which an intercostal approach was used, local analgesic blockade of the intercostal nerves located two spaces either side of the surgical site using a long acting agent, such as bupivacaine, provides effective pain relief (Berg and Orton, 1986). Other regional analgesic techniques have been described by Hall and Clark (1984).

SPECIAL CONSIDERATIONS

Central nervous system trauma

The need for an anaesthetic agent to produce unconsciousness and analgesia should be ascertained before administering drugs to patients with nervous system injury. Comatose patients may not require any anaesthetic agents. In other patients, diazepam may be administered as a premedicant with or without a lose dose of an opioid agent (Shapiro, 1986a). For induction of anaesthesia, thiobarbiturates are preferred for cardiovascularly stable patients since they are considered to have 'protective' effects against hypoxic neuronal damage and will lower ICP and cerebral blood flow (Bedford and Durbin, 1986). Isoflurane has been advocated as the inhalational agent of choice because it causes less cerebral vasodilatation than halothane or enflurane (Cucchiara, Theye and

Michenfelder, 1974; Michenfelder, 1984). Halothane may be satisfactory when combined with hyperventilation. Anaesthetic agents which significantly increase ICP, such as ketamine, are best avoided. Fluid administration should restore normal hydration without overhydration. Dextrose-containing solutions should not be used because hyperglycaemia may enhance post-ischaemic neurological damage (Welsh, Gensberg and Rieder, 1980). Large volumes of lactated Ringer's solution may also cause problems since this solution is relatively hypo-osmolar and may increase ICP in patients that have received osmotic diuretics (Todd *et al.*, 1984). An iso-osmotic solution such as normal saline has been cited as the preferred crystalloid volume replacement solution (Domino, 1987). Once deficits have been replaced the recommended fluid administration rate is 1–2 ml kg^{-1} h^{-1}. Head trauma patients should be monitored closely for ventilatory impairment in the recovery period.

Ocular trauma

When anaesthetizing patients with ocular trauma, precautions must be taken to avoid raising intraocular pressure (IOP) such that eyeball rupture does not occur. Accordingly, ketamine and suxamethonium (succinylcholine) should not be employed since these agents are known to increase IOP significantly (Adams, 1982).

Cardiac trauma

Traumatic myocarditis and cardiac tamponade may occur following trauma. The exact incidence of traumatic myocarditis in the veterinary patient population is unclear but it has been described as frequent with the highest incidence in large breed dogs (Alexander, Bolton and Koslow, 1975; Macintire and Snider, 1984). Traumatic myocarditis occurs as a direct result of thoracic injury or indirectly when the neural or vascular supply to the heart is damaged. A patient may be presented with normal cardiovascular function and subsequently develop cardiac dysrhythmias within 12–48 hours of the traumatic insult (Buffum and Dodd, 1978; Macintire and Snider, 1984). Commonly observed dysrhythmias are premature ventricular depolarizations, ventricular tachycardia, sinus tachycardia and atrial fibrillation (Alexander *et al.*, 1975; Madewell, Nelson and Hill, 1977; Macintire and Snider, 1984). Attempts should be made to resolve dysrhythmias preoperatively. When a patient has to be anaesthetized before the cardiac rhythm disturbance can be resolved, the anaesthetic protocol should be designed to minimize depression of cardiac contractility and agents which are less likely to aggravate the dysrhythmia should be employed. In this respect, low doses of acepromazine or an opioid agent are satisfactory for premedication and isoflurane is a suitable agent for induction and maintenance of anaesthesia. Antidys-rhythmic therapy should be continued throughout the operative period and into the recovery period if necessary.

Cardiac tamponade may occur in association with haemopericar-dium. Diastolic filling of the heart is impaired and CO becomes dependent on heart rate. Pericardiocentesis should be attempted preoperatively to improve CO and the anaesthetic regimen should avoid causing bradycardia and severe depression of myocardial contractility.

Ruptured mitral valves have been noted following trauma (Kaplan, 1987). The anaesthetic management of these cases is similar to that described for mitral insufficiency (Seeler *et al.*, 1988).

Abdominal trauma

Rupture of the liver or spleen. The liver and spleen have been reported to be the most commonly injured abdominal organs following trauma (Carb, 1974; Ewing, 1975). Rupture of either organ may be associated with massive blood loss into the abdomi-nal cavity. Aggressive shock therapy and monitoring is required and blood transfusion is often necessary. The anaesthetic protocol should cause minimal cardiovascular depression. Phenothiazines should be avoided in favour of opioid agents or neuroleptanalgesic combinations when sedation or analgesia is required. Induction of anaesthesia or narcosis with a volatile agent or opioid agent with subsequent maintenance of anaesthesia using an inhalational agent is the authors' preferred technique. Barbiturates should be avoided in patients with splenic trauma because they cause splenic engorgement and may exacerbate hypotension by causing a sudden decrease in vasomotor tone. Furthermore, removal of an engorged spleen will significantly diminish the blood volume of the patient. When the abdomen is opened and intra-abdominal pressure relieved, an episode of acute hypostatic hypotension may occur. The anaesthetist can prepare for this event by fluid-loading the patient and by ensuring that a suitable vasoconstrictor is available.

Trauma of the urinary tract. In a survey of animals injured in automobile accidents, damage to the renal system occurred more frequently than damage to any other abdominal organ system (Kolata and Johnston, 1975). Sixty-two per cent of animals with renal system damage had a ruptured bladder, 20% had a ruptured ureter or urethra, and 13% had a ruptured kidney. Most instances of trauma to the urinary system are not life-threatening and the patient often can be stabilized prior to anaesthesia. Exceptions include cases with avulsion of the renal pedicle or when there is extensive fragmentation of the kidney. These conditions are often associated with massive haemorrhage or even sudden death. Such patients should be managed as previously described for patients in shock.

Rupture of the urinary tract is often accompanied by uraemia, hyperkalaemia, hyponatraemia and hypochloraemia. Preanaesthetic stabilization of these patients involves infusion of 2.5% dextrose with 0.45% sodium chloride to correct the electrolyte imbalance and any fluid deficits. A urethral catheter may be inserted to pass through the rupture into the peritoneum to drain abdominal fluid. If this is unsuccessful, peritoneal dialysis may be instituted (Archibald *et al.*, 1981). Once the patient has been stabilized, anaesthesia should progress routinely, although agents which require extensive renal clearance to terminate their action (ketamine, gallamine) should be avoided.

Trauma of the gastrointestinal tract. Reports of gastrointestinal injury, although rare, may occur as a result of penetrating wounds and blunt blows which cause thrombosis, avulsion or torsion of the blood supply to the intestine (Parker and Presnell, 1972; Archibald and Sumner-Smith, 1974). Septic shock must be suspected in such patients (Ledingham and McArdle, 1978). Treatment of patients with septic shock has been outlined elsewhere (Crowe, 1985). It may include administration of flunixin meglumine and corticosteroids to alleviate some of the negative circulatory effects of endotoxins (Hardie and Rawlings, 1983). A potassium–dextrose–insulin mixture may be administered intravenously to relieve the energy crisis induced by septic shock (Crowe, 1985). An intravenous infusion of dopamine or dobutamine can be used to support cardiac output.

Orthopaedic trauma

Most cases of orthopaedic trauma do not require immediate surgery and should undergo thorough preoperative assessment and stabilization. Specific problems which may be encountered in these patients include extensive blood loss from the fracture site, particularly in animals with femoral fractures, and hyperkalaemia resulting from extensive tissue damage.

Premedication, induction and maintenance of anaesthesia do not need to vary substantially from standard protocols once cardiopulmonary stability is established. Preoperative use of an opioid agent to provide analgesia and allay apprehension is desirable. Intraoperative analgesia may be enhanced by intravenous administration of an opioid agent or by irrigation of the fractured ends of long bones with a local anaesthetic agent. The latter technique is particularly useful for reduction of rib fractures (Hall and Clark, 1984). Intraoperative blood loss may be significant, notably during repair of maxillary or pelvic fractures. The volume of blood loss should be closely monitored and replaced.

Postoperative analgesia is an important consideration in orthopaedic cases. Opioid analgesic agents are of value for this purpose and are best administered before the return of consciousness. Lumbosacral epidural administration of an epidural preparation of morphine (0.1 mg kg^{-1}), bupivacaine (0.5% at 1 ml 4.5 kg^{-1}) or mepivacaine (2.0% at 1 ml 4.5 kg^{-1}) have been used safely to provide several hours of postoperative analgesia in dogs (Bonath and Saleh, 1985; Heath *et al.*, 1985).

Burns

Animals with extensive burns are occasionally encountered in veterinary practice. Specific problems which may affect these patients include pain, cardiovascular depression, a hypermetabolic state, loss of body heat, sepsis, glottic oedema, and gastrointestinal bleeding (Lamb, 1985). There is no entirely satisfactory method of pain relief for burn victims. Systemic administration of opioid agents may ease acute pain and low doses of ketamine have been reported to provide effective pain relief in man (Lamb, 1985). The latter technique, however, is associated with the risk of airway obstruction.

Peripheral circulatory failure is mediated by vasoactive agents which cause increased capillary permeability throughout the body (Moncrief, 1973). Large quantities of intravascular fluid, electrolytes and plasma proteins are lost to the extravascular space and a reduction in cardiac output and pulmonary oedema may result. Interstitial fluid volume is also severely reduced by transfer of fluid into the cells of injured tissues (Moncrief, 1973). Most fluid translocation occurs within 12 hours of the time of injury and normal capillary permeability is restored after 24 hours (Moncrief, 1973). Myocardial depressant factors such as interleukins and complement released from burn injuries have been implicated in reducing myocardial function (Moncrief, 1973). Aggressive monitoring and therapy of the fluid volume status of the patient with burns is required. The generalized increase in capillary permeability lasts for approximately 24 hours and it has been suggested that during this time only crystalloid solutions be administered at 10 ml kg^{-1} h^{-1} (Moncrief, 1973; De Campo and Aldrete, 1981). Colloid solutions may be introduced after this period. Burn injuries may induce haemolysis, reduce red cell survival time and microthrom-boembolism (Cullen, 1986). Débridement of burn wounds often results in significant haemorrhage, and blood transfusions may be required (Lamb, 1985).

A hypermetabolic state begins within hours of the burn injury and persists until the wounds heal (Wilmore and Aulick, 1978). Consequently, there is an increased rate of catabolism, increased oxygen utilization, increased carbon dioxide production, hyper-thermia, and hyperglycaemia. The degree of increase in the metabolic rate is proportional to the size of the burn (Lamb, 1985). It is mediated by increased adrenergic activity and an endogenous resetting of energy production (Boutros and Hoyt, 1976). The metabolic rate and associated patient stress can be reduced by increasing the temperature of the environment to approximately 34°C (Moncrief, 1973).

Hypothermia results from significant evaporative losses from large areas of exposed surface and adds to patient stress. Exposed body surfaces should be covered, the room heated and intravenous fluids warmed. Glottic oedema may follow inhalation of steam, smoke and other toxic substances and cause airway obstruction or make intubation difficult (Lamb, 1985). Sepsis is due to loss of the protective epidermal barrier, impairment of the immune system and the presence of avascular burned tissue which provides a good culture medium. Suitable antibiotic therapy should be initiated (Cullen, 1986). Gastrointestinal bleeding may occur as a result of gastric or duodenal mucosal ischaemia (Cullen, 1986).

The selection of anaesthetic agents for burn patients is not critical if it is performed on a rational basis. Barbiturates should not be used in hypovolaemic patients. Incorporation of opioid agents into the anaesthetic protocol is desirable because of their analgesic properties and their ability to reduce the requirement for inhalational anaesthetic agents. All inhalational agents are suitable. Adequate arterial oxygenation should be ensured before administering nitrous oxide, because oxygen consumption and pulmonary shunt fraction are often increased in burn patients.

An abnormal response to muscle relaxants has been noted in human burn victims. Sensitivity to suxamethonium (succinylcho-line) is increased in proportion to the size of the burn (Tolmie, 1967). Large quantities of potassium are released into the circulation and cardiac arrest may result (Tolmie, 1967). The risk of this occurring is greatest in the period of 5 days to 3 months after the injury is sustained (Gronert and Theye, 1975). The mechanism of increased sensitivity is unknown but may involve an increased number of post-junctional receptors (Gronert and Theye, 1975). In contrast, resistance to non-depolarizing muscle relaxants is increased by a factor of 1.5–2 in patients with greater than 25% of the body surface area affected (Leibel, 1981; Martyn *et al.*, 1984). The period of abnormal response is equivalent to that for suxamethonium.

REFERENCES

Adams, H. R. (1982). In *Veterinary Pharmacology and Therapeutics*, 5th edn, p. 144, eds. N. H. Booth & L. E. McDonald. Ames, Iowa: Iowa State University Press.

Alexander, J. W., Bolton, G. R. and Koslow, G. L. (1975). *Journal of the American Animal Hospital Association* 11, 160.

Archibald, J. and Sumner-Smith, G. (1974). In *Canine Surgery*, ed. J. Archibald. Santa Barbara: American Veterinary Publications.

Archibald, J., Holt, J. C. and Sokolovsky, V. (1981). In *Management of Trauma in Dogs and Cats*, ed. E. J. Catcott, p. 64. Santa Barbara: American Veterinary Publications.

Bedford, R. F. and Durbin, C. G. (1986). In *Anesthesia*, ed. R. D. Miller, p. 2253. New York: Churchill Livingstone.

Berg, R. J. and Orton, E. C. (1986). *American Journal of Veterinary Research*, 47, 471.

Berkwitt, L. and Berzon, J. L. (1985). *Veterinary Clinics of North America: Small Animal Practice* 15 (5), 1031.

Bonath, K. H. and Saleh, A. S. (1985). *Proceedings of the 2nd International Congress of Veterinary Anesthesia* 161.

Bond, A. C. and Davis, C. K. (1974). *Anesthesia* 29, 59.

Booth, N. H. (1982). In *Veterinary Pharmacology and Therapeutics*, 5th edn, p. 241, eds. N. H. Booth and L. E. McDonald. Ames, Iowa: Iowa State University Press.

Boutros, A. R. and Hoyt, J. R. (1976). *Critical Care Medicine* 4, 144.

Buffum, R. M. and Dodd, R. R. (1978). *Canine Practice* 5 (5), 30.

Carb, A. V. (1974). *Veterinary Surgery* 3, 19.

Chasapakis, G., Kekis, N., Sakklais, C. and Kolios, D. (1973). *Anesthesia and Analgesia* 52,282.

Child, K. J., Currie, J. P., Davis, B., Dodds, M. G., Pearce, D. R. and Twissell, D. J. (1971). *British Journal of Anaesthesia* 43, 2.

Clark, D. R. (1982). In *Veterinary Pharmacology and Therapeutics*, 5th edn, p. 503, eds. N. H. Booth and L. E. McDonald. Ames, Iowa: Iowa State University Press.

Clarke, R. S. J. and Carson, I. W. (1980). In *General Anaesthesia*, eds. T. C. Gray, J. F. Nunn and J. E. Utting, p. 1297. Boston: Butterworths & Co.

Corbett, H. R. (1976). *Australian Veterinary Practitioner* 6, 147.

Court, M. H., Dodman, N. H. and Seeler, D. C. (1985). *Veterinary Clinics of North America* 15 (5), 1041.

Crowe, D. T. (1985). *Journal of Veterinary Critical Care* 8 (1), 7.

Cucchiara, R. F., Theye, R. A. and Michenfelder, J. D. (1974). *Anesthesiology* **40**, 571.

Cullen, B. F. (1986). *37th Annual Refresher Course Lectures of the ASA (Oct.)* 176.

Davis, L. E. (1984). In *Veterinary Trauma and Critical Care*, ed. I. M. Zaslow, p. 287. Philadelphia: Lea & Febiger.

De Campo, T. and Aldrete, J. A. (1981). *Intensive Care Medicine* **7**, 55.

Dodman, N. H. (1980). *Veterinary Record* **107**, 481.

Dodman, N. H., Seeler, D. C. and Court, M. H. (1984). *British Veterinary Journal* **140**, 505.

Domino, K. B. (1987). *37th Annual Refresher Course Lectures of the A5A (Oct.)* 175.

Douglas, M. E., Downs, J. B., Dannemiller, E. J. and Hodges, M. R. (1976). *Surgery, Gynecology and Obstetrics* **143**, 555.

Eger, E. I. (1974). In *Anesthetic Uptake and Action*, p. 134. Baltimore, New York: Williams & Wilkins.

Eger, E. I. II, Saidman, L. J. and Brandstater, B. (1965). *Anesthesiology* **28**, 756.

Ewing, G. D. (1975). *Canine Practice* **2** (4), 22.

Fishman, A. P. (1981). *New England Journal of Medicine* **304** (9), 537.

Freeman, J. and Nunn, J. F. (1963). *Clinical Sciences* **24**, 135.

Garson, H. L., Dodman, N. H. and Baker, G. J. (1980). *Journal of Small Animal Practice* **20** (9), 469.

Graves, C. L. (1974). *International Anesthesiology Clinics* **12** (1), 16.

Gronert, G. A. and Theye, R. A. (1975). *Anesthesiology* **43**, 89.

Guyton, A. C. (1986). In *Textbook of Medical Physiology*, p. 327. Philadelphia: W. B. Saunders Company.

Halford, F. J. (1943). *Anesthesiology* **4**, 67.

Hall, L. W. and Clark, K. W. (1984). In *Veterinary Anaesthesia*, p. 183. London: Baillière Tindall.

Hardie, E. M. and Rawlings, C. A. (1983). *Compendium of Continuing Education for the Practicing Veterinarian* **5**, 483.

Haskins, S. C. (1981). *American Journal of Veterinary Research* **42** (5), 856.

Haskins, S. C. (1984). In *Veterinary Trauma and Critical Care*, ed. I. M. Zaslow, p. 339. Philadelphia: Lea & Febiger.

Haskins, S. (1987). In *Principles and Practice of Veterinary Anesthesia*, ed. C. Short, p. 455. Baltimore, New York: Williams and Wilkins.

Heath, R. B., Broadstone, R. V., Wright, M. and Grandy, J. (1985). *Proceedings of the 2nd International Congress of Veterinary Anesthesia* 162.

Henning, R. (1986). *Anaesthesia and Intensive Care* **14**, 267.

Hickey, R. F. and Eger, E. I. (1986). In *Anesthesia*, ed. R. D. Miller, p. 651. New York: Churchill Livingstone.

Hoelzer, M. F. (1986). *Emergency Medicine Clinics of North America* **4** (3), 487.

Kaplan, P. J. (1987). Personal communication.

Kernodle, D. S., DiRaimondo, C. R. and Fulkerson, W. J. (1984). *South Medical Journal* **77**, 318.

Kirkwood, C. G., Edwards, D. J., Lalka, D., Lasezkay, G., Hassett, J. M. and Slaughter, R. L. (1986). *Journal of Trauma* **26** (12), 1090.

Kolata, R. J. (1981). In *Management of Trauma in Dogs and Cats*, ed. E. J. Catcott, p. 11. Santa Barbara: American Veterinary Publications.

Kolata, R. J. and Johnson, D. E. (1975). *Journal of the American Veterinary Medical Association* **167**, 938.

Kolata, R. J. and Rawlings, C. A. (1982). *Journal of the American Animal Hospital Association* **43**, 2196.

Kolata, R. J., Kraut, N. H. and Johnson, D. E. (1973). *Journal of the American Veterinary Medical Association* **164**, 449.

Lamb, J. D. (1985). *Canadian Anaesthetists Society Journal* **32**, 84.

Lanning, C. F. and Harmel, M. H. (1975). *Annual Review of Medicine* **26**, 137.

Ledingham, I. McA. and McArdle, C. S. (1978). *Lancet* **ii**, 470.

Leibel, W. S. (1981). *Anesthesiology* **54**, 378.

Macintire, D. K. and Snider, T. G. (1984). *Journal of the American Veterinary Medical Association* **184** (5), 541.

Madewell, B. R., Nelson, D. T. and Hill, K. (1977). *Journal of the American Veterinary Medical Association* **171**, 273.

Mahafan, V. K., Simon, M. and Huber, G. L. (1979). *Chest* **75**, 192.

Markoo, A. K. (1986). *Annals of Emergency Medicine* **15**, 1470.

Marshall, B. E. (1986). *37th Annual Refresher Course Lectures of the ASA (Oct.)* 146.

Martyn, J. A. J., Matted, R. S., Szylelbsein, S. K. and Kaplan, R. F. (1984). *Anesthesia and Analgesia* **61**, 614.

Massion, W. H. (1974). *International Anesthesiology Clinics* **12** (1), 223.

McIntosh, T. K. and Faden, A. I. (1986). *Annals of Emergency Medicine* **15** (12), 1462.

Michenfelder, J. D. (1984). *35th Annual Refresher Course Lectures of the ASA (Oct.)* 118.

Miller, R. D. (1986). *International Anesthesia Research Society Review Course Lectures* 89.

Moncrief, J. A. (1973). *New England Journal of Medicine* **288**, 444.

Parker, W. M. and Presnell, K. R. (1972). *Canadian Veterinary Journal* **13**, 282.

Pascoe, P. J. (1987). In *Principles and Practice of Veterinary Anesthesia*, ed. C. Short, p. 558. Baltimore, New York: Williams and Wilkins.

Priano, L. L. (1985). *Anesthesiology* **63**, 357.

Raffe, M. R. (1987). In *Principles and Practice of Veterinary Anesthesia*, ed. C. Short, p. 478. Baltimore, New York: Williams and Wilkins.

Ray, R. J., Alexander, C. M., Chen, L., Williams, J. and Marshall, B. E. (1984). *Critical Care Medicine* **12**, 364.

Savarese, J. J. (1986). *International Anesthesia Research Society Review Course Lectures* 90.

Savino, J. L. and Del Guercio, L. R. M. (1985). *Surgical Clinics of North America* **65** (4), 763.

Seeler, D. C., Dodman, N. H., Norman, W. M. and Court, M. H. (1988). *British Veterinary Journal* **144**, 108.

Seyde, W. C. and Longnecker, D. E. (1984). *Anesthesiology* **61**, 686.

Shapiro, H. M. (1986a). In *Anesthesia*, ed. R. D. Miller, p. 1600. New York: Churchill Livingstone.

Shapiro, H. M. (1986b). In *Anesthesia*, ed. R. D. Miller, p. 2215. New York: Churchill Livingstone.

Smith, D. S. (1987). *38th Annual Refresher Course Lectures of the ASA (Oct.)* 521.

Spence, A. (1980). In *General Anaesthesia*, eds T. C. Gray, J. F. Nunn and J. E. Utting, p. 591. Boston: Butterworths.

Tamas, P., Paddleford, R. R. and Krahwinkle, D. J. (1983). *Scientific Session. American College of Veterinary Anesthesiologists* 1.

Todd, M. M., Tommasino, C., Moore, S. and Drummond, J. C. (1984). *Anesthesiology* **61**, A122.

Tolmie, J. D. (1967). *Anesthesiology* **28**, 467.

Traber, D. L., Wilson, R. D. and Priano, L. L. (1968). *Anesthesia and Analgesia* **47**, 769.

Weiskopf, R. B., Townsley, M. I. and Riordan, K. K. (1981). *Anesthesia and Analgesia* **60**, 481.

Welsh, F. A., Gensberg, M. D. and Rieder, W. (1980). *Stroke* **11**, 355.

Wilmore, D. W. and Aulick, L. H. (1978). *Surgical Clinics of North America* **58**, 1173.

Wilson, R. F., Larned, P. A., Corr, J. J., Sarver, E. J. and Barrett, D. M. (1970). *Journal of Surgery Research* **10**, 571.

4

Anaesthesia for patients with respiratory insufficiency

Of all the disease conditions which may be detected prior to anaesthesia, there is none so threatening as those which affect either cardiac or respiratory function. Patients may be physiologically compensated and asymptomatic at rest, but will have reduced cardiac or pulmonary reserve making them more vulnerable to general anaesthesia.

The account which follows considers measures that can be used to minimize this risk. The successful management of anaesthesia in patients with coincident respiratory disease requires: (1) an accurate diagnosis of the disorder; (2) an understanding of the physiological disturbances which result; (3) the appreciation and application of measures which will improve the patient's condition prior to and following anaesthesia; (4) a working knowledge of the relevant pharmacology of anaesthetic agents, and (5) appropriate selection of anaesthetic technique to minimize the impact of anaesthesia on the disease process.

PREOPERATIVE EVALUATION

History

The most obvious indications of respiratory insufficiency include coughing, exercise intolerance, or dyspnoea at rest or after exercise. These may be indicative of a significant cardiac or pulmonary disorder and warrant a comprehensive clinical examination of the patient. Cyanosis is a grave prognostic sign which indicates severe pathophysiological changes and also signifies poor anaesthetic risk potential.

53

Clinical examination

The rate, depth, and nature of respiration should be determined in every patient prior to anaesthesia. Often, rapid, shallow or irregular breathing is the first indication of a respiratory problem. In severe cases of respiratory distress, laboured breathing or paradoxical movements of the thoracic wall and abdomen are usually obvious. Animals may stand with their elbows abducted and may be mouth breathing when the condition is this severe.

A vital part of clinical examination of the respiratory system is the evaluation of the adequacy of the airway. This involves inspection of the oropharynx and upper respiratory tract. The buccal cavity, pharynx and laryngeal aditus should also be inspected by direct vision, using a laryngoscope if necessary, to determine whether potentially obstructive lesions are present. It is also important to palpate the retropharyngeal area and trachea to check for unusual luminal or extraluminal structures which may cause compression or stenosis of the airway. Digital compression of the trachea to induce a cough is a useful manoeuvre which may be used to distinguish tracheitis from other conditions which cause coughing.

Clinical evaluation of the lungs themselves usually involves auscultation. This helps to identify the type, distribution and degree of any pulmonary lesions. The technique does, however, require practice to distinguish subtle alterations in the normally phasic inspiratory and expiratory flow patterns (Kotlikoff and Gillespie, 1984). Gross disturbances in flow resulting in continuous turbulence are easier to discern and are indicative of severe pulmonary structural change, or flow pattern changes (Kotlikoff and Gillespie, 1983). Occasionally, tracheal auscultation is useful to evaluate the flow pattern when breathing is quiet. It can also help to distinguish abnormal upper respiratory sounds from those generated within the lungs themselves. If pulmonary disease is suspected, percussion of the chest wall will help to identify areas of consolidation and the presence of fluid or gas within the pleural space. Palpation of the apex beat will establish whether the normal topographical relationship exists between the heart and the lungs.

Evaluation of the cardiorespiratory system after exercise is an important aspect of thorough clinical examination as some conditions which are compensated at rest only become apparent following exercise.

Ancillary diagnostic tests

Radiography. Lateral and dorsoventral radiographs are valuable in the diagnosis and quantification of intrathoracic lesions. Care should be taken when radiographing animals which are in respiratory distress because inappropriate positioning can worsen their condition. It is advisable to take standing lateral views and dorsoventral views in these patients rather than risk the struggling and positional dyspnoea sometimes associated with lateral or dorsal recumbency. The cardiac silhouette should be evaluated when interpreting thoracic radiographs as left-sided heart failure resulting in pulmonary oedema, or right-sided heart enlargement secondary to pulmonary disease (cor pulmonale), may be detected in some dyspnoeic patients.

Blood gas analysis. If facilities are available, arterial blood gas analysis should be performed preoperatively in every case of suspected moderate to severe respiratory insufficiency. The analysis of blood gases will indicate whether respiratory gas transfer is normal and which patients are significantly compromised. The normal partial pressure of oxygen in arterial blood (Pao_2) when room air is respired is 85–100 mmHg in the dog, and 78–100 mmHg in the cat. The normal partial pressure of carbon dioxide in arterial blood ($Paco_2$) is 29–42 mmHg in both dog and cat (Tasker, 1980).

Pulmonary function tests. These were designed for use in humans and most of these tests require the voluntary cooperation of the patient. However, one test which can be used in animals is the measurement of tidal volume (V_T) or minute respiratory volume (MRV) using a face mask and a hand-held respirometer. The tidal volume for small animal patients is normally 10–20 ml kg^{-1} and the MRV is 150–250 ml kg^{-1} min^{-1} (Haskins, 1983; Hall and Clarke, 1983). An estimate of alveolar ventilation can be made if it is assumed that the dead space volume (V_D) per breath is 25–33% of the tidal volume.

$$\text{Alveolar ventilation} = (V_T - V_D) \times \text{respiratory rate}$$

Alveolar ventilation of 100–130 ml kg^{-1} min^{-1} is usually adequate to maintain eucapnia. When ventilation–perfusion imbalance exists, however, even this level of ventilation may prove inadequate to maintain a normal Pao_2 (hypoxaemic respiratory insufficiency). If the measued MRV or estimated alveolar ventilation is below normal, the patient is hypoventilating and hypoxia and hypercapnia will be present simultaneously (combined hypoxaemic/hypercapnic respiratory insufficiency). The normal physiological response to increasing carbon dioxide levels is hyperventilation, or at least an increased ventilatory effort. It should be remembered that although hyperventilation is frequently observed in patients with pulmonary disorders, it may also be a result of metabolic acidosis, fear, pain or fever. Under these circumstances the $Paco_2$ is usually low.

Significance of conditions found

When a patient is found to have respiratory insufficiency, it is important to make a definitive diagnosis of the disease condition. The anaesthetic management of individual cases may differ according to the type of respiratory disturbance present. In general, respiratory disorders may be divided into two major categories.

Extrapulmonary conditions. These primarily affect pulmonary ventilation (Table 1). Each disease process has its own specific treatment and prognosis, but general principles can be applied which will improve the condition of the patient. Some conditions will respond to medical therapy and may be partially resolved prior to surgery, others may be intractable or even progressive. Severe obstructive lesions can sometimes be bypassed by tracheotomy prior to anaesthesia, while certain extrapulmonary restrictive disorders can be ameliorated by positional change or by use of techniques such as paracentesis.

Pulmonary conditions. These affect alveolar ventilation, pulmonary blood flow or the normal ventilation–perfusion balance within the lung (Table 2). If medical treatment is unsuccessful, or if time does not permit resolution of the lesion, there are no definitive surgical measures which can improve the condition of the patient. Specific pharmacological agents given preoperatively may be palliative in some cases. Pulmonary conditions are often more sinister than the more dramatic extrapulmonary lesions because of their refractoriness. In patients with ventilation to perfusion mismatch, pulmonary ventilation and cardiac output must be maintained and additional derangements of ventilation/perfusion balance avoided if at all possible.

It is not only the type of respiratory disturbance which determines the management of patients with respiratory insufficiency, but also the degree of respiratory impairment. Mild respiratory distubances may only require minor modification of anaesthetic protocol, but when respiratory failure is present a re-evaluation of patient management is required. The latter patients benefit best from 'maximal support techniques' (Milledge and Nunn, 1980). An arbitrary, but useful, classification of the degree of respiratory disturbance is as follows:

Table 1. Extrapulmonary causes of ventilatory impairment

Obstructive	*Restrictive*
Larynx:	*Intrapleural:*
Hypoplasia	Diaphragmatic hernia
Stenosis (stricture, web)	Hydrothorax, haemothorax, chylothorax, pyothorax
Oedema	Pneumothorax
Spasm	
Foreign body	*Thoracic wall:*
Neoplasia	Kyphosis, lordosis
Everted lateral ventricles	Pectus excavatum
Extralaryngeal mass (retropharyngeal abscess)	Flail chest
	Neoplasia
Subepiglottic cyst	Body bandages
Collapsed arytenoids	Obesity
Laryngeal paralysis	
	Abdominal:
Trachea:	Ascites
Stenosis	Neoplasia
Hypoplasia	Haemoperitoneum
Collapse	Gastric dilatation (bloat)
Foreign body	
Oedema	
Neoplasia	
Filaroides osleri (dog)	

Mild: No obvious respiratory problems at rest. Condition only diagnosed by careful clinical examination and by the use of ancillary diagnostic techniques.

Moderate: Hypopnoea, tachypnoea or cough readily apparent at rest, but well tolerated by the patient. Obviously altered upper airway or pulmonary sounds apparent on auscultation. Ancillary diagnostic tests confirm a derangement in function.

Severe: Dyspnoea with or without cyanosis at rest. Condition is potentially life-threatening. If the Pao_2 is below 60 mmHg when the patient is breathing air, or the $Paco_2$ is above 46 mmHg, the patient should be considered to be in respiratory failure (Snyder, 1973).

Table 2. Pulmonary causes of ventilatory impairment and ventilation–perfusion mismatch

Obstructive	Restrictive	Ventilation–perfusion mismatch
Excessive secretions	Pulmonary neoplasia	Pulmonary contusion
Bronchitis	Bullous neoplasia	Pneumonia
Filaroides osleri (dog)	Pulmonary contusion	Pulmonary neoplasia
Allergic asthma	Hyaline membrane disease	Pulmonary embolism
Pulmonary oedema	Pneumonia	*Aelurostrongylus abstrusus* (cat)
	Pulmonary oedema Infiltrative disease	*Dirofilaria immitis* (dog)

PREOPERATIVE PREPARATION

In keeping with requirements for safe anaesthetic practice, the condition of animals with respiratory insufficiency should be improved as far as possible before anaesthesia and surgery. Appropriate preparation of these patients will help to circumvent acute problems and may reduce the incidence of postoperative complications. When surgery is for alleviating respiratory impairment, temporary or palliative measures are necessary preoperatively to reduce anaesthetic risk. The delay which preoperative preparation necessitates is often well compensated in terms of reduced postoperative morbidity and mortality and is, of course, in the best interests of the patient. When surgery is vital and pressing, however, the optimum time to operate is necessarily a compromise.

Oxygen. Oxygen supplementation is often indicated preoperatively for patients with respiratory disorders (Haskins, 1983). Exceptions include patients with mild forms of respiratory impairment, and those in which the hypoxic drive to ventilation is crucial (West, 1982). Oxygen can be administered via a nasal tube or face mask, but is probably better administered by means of an oxygen cage (Court, Dodman and Seeler, 1985). The percentage of oxygen required varies for each patient and is best determined by measurement of the Pao_2 (Fitzpatrick and Crowe, 1986; Haskins, 1983). In the absence of facilities for arterial blood gas analysis, it may be necessary to check the colour of the oral or palpebral mucous membranes, or to administer the maximum percentage of oxygen attainable by the method of oxygen administration employed.

Whatever method is selected, it is recommended that oxygen delivered to the patient is humidified by bubbling it through a heated humidifier or nebulizer to prevent desiccation of the respiratory mucosa (Court, Dodman and Seeler, 1985; Fitzpatrick and Crowe, 1986; McKiernan, 1983).

Surgical interventions. A tracheotomy can be performed under local anaesthesia prior to general anaesthesia and is indicated in patients with severe extrapulmonary obstructive disease involving the larynx or upper trachea. The use of neuroleptanalgesic combinations may be necessary to calm a distressed patient and facilitate the insertion of the tracheostomy tube. The technique for performing a tracheotomy is described elsewhere (Aron and Crowe, 1985).

Paracentesis should be performed preoperatively in patients with moderate to severe extrapulmonary restrictive disease resulting from an accumulation of air or fluid within the pleural or peritoneal cavities. Respiratory distress can often be significantly alleviated in this way. In most instances, paracentesis can be performed easily under local anaesthesia using a trochar and catheter. After insertion, the catheter is sutured in place and attached to a large syringe or vacuum source by means of a three-way tap. If large volumes of fluid or blood are withdrawn rapidly from either cavity, there is risk of circulatory collapse (Hartsfield, 1985) so cardiovascular function should be monitored. It is often necessary to infuse a crystalloid solution, plasma volume replacement solution, or whole blood in order to maintain an effective circulating blood volume. The measurement of central venous pressure can be extremely valuable in determining the correct volume of the replacement solution to be administered.

Chemotherapy

Antibiotics. Bacterial pneumonias and other bacterial respiratory disorders should be treated with broad-spectrum antibiotics prior to anaesthesia to reduce pulmonary risk factors and minimize postoperative pulmonary complications (Marsh, 1983).

Diuretics. Conditions which may benefit from diuretic therapy preoperatively include pulmonary oedema and viral pneumonias (Raffin, 1982). These conditions have both an obstructive and restrictive component and will cause ventilation–perfusion imbalance. Diuresis will decrease lung water and improve pulmonary gas exchange. This therapy can worsen the condition of patients with purulent conditions by increasing the viscosity of already thick secretions and so should probably not be performed in such cases (Raffin, 1982).

Bronchodilators. Patients with pulmonary disease in which there is obstruction to airflow are likely to benefit from treatment with bronchodilators prior to anaesthesia. Bronchodilators which can be used include methylxanthines, such as aminophylline, and the β_2-adrenergic drugs, such as terbutaline. Anticholinergics, such as atropine, may also be useful on occasion since they reduce cholinergic bronchoconstriction, but it should be remembered that these agents also cause drying of secretions.

Antihistamines. In man, antihistamines are useful therapeutic agents for alleviating the histamine-mediated component of bronchial asthma (Hirshman, 1981). Although bronchial asthma does occur in the cat (Moses and Spaulding, 1985), it appears that the chemical mediators are different and antihistamines are probably of little or no value (Spaulding, 1987). Clinical cases of asthma have not been reported in the dog although it is known that some dogs have naturally-acquired bronchial reaginic activity (Frick, 1974).

Steroids. Bronchoconstriction associated with feline asthma can also be obtunded using steroids (Moses and Spaulding, 1985). These agents are also valuable in minimizing the tissue reaction associated with traumatic pulmonary disease such as pulmonary contusion, pulmonary barotrauma and smoke inhalation (Tams and Sherding, 1981). Rapidly-acting water-soluble steroids—e.g., prednisolone sodium succinate or dexamethasone phosphate—provide the most immediate effect.

PREMEDICATION

No firm rules can be made regarding the selection of premedicant drugs for patients with respiratory insufficiency. Agents should be chosen which are appropriate for the pathophysiological state of the animal. They should be administered for the purpose of calming anxious or nervous patients, facilitating anaesthetic induction and maintenance, and making the procedure safer and more comfortable for the patient (Hall, 1971). An essential prerequisite in the selection of preanaesthetic agents is that they should not aggravate the respiratory condition and should not depress cardiovascular function excessively. In some instances, premedication may actually improve the animal's condition and make breathing easier. To some extent, the choice of agent will depend on the anaesthetic technique which is to follow.

Sedative agents, such as acepromazine, are relatively safe to use in patients with mild respiratory conditions, but they should be avoided when there is preoperative CO_2 retention or when the

Pao_2 is low. This is because most sedatives depress the responsiveness of the central nervous system to CO_2 and hypoxia (Fairley, 1981). Sedative agents should also be avoided in patients with extrapulmonary obstructive disease because relaxation of pharyngeal muscle tone may contribute to the obstruction and exacerbate the condition. In the canine brachycephalic airway syndrome (which has many features in common with the human sleep apnoea syndrome) induction of a sleep-like state or anaesthesia may contribute to the development of obstructive apnoea (Amis and Kurpershoek, 1986). For this reason, the authors avoid the use of acepromazine in brachycephalic dogs.

Opioid agents, such as morphine, can be useful for the premedication of dogs with mild respiratory insufficiency, particularly if anxiolysis or analgesia is desirable. However, certain limitations should be borne in mind regarding the use of these agents. First, it should be remembered that opioid drugs are potent ventilatory depressants (Hall and Clarke, 1983) and as such they should be used cautiously when respiratory disorders are present. Paradoxically, however, in patients with pulmonary oedema some opioid analgesics can modify rapid and shallow respirations to a deeper and more effective pattern and will also reduce pulmonary capillary pressure by diverting blood from the pulmonary circuit (Davis, 1979). Second, most opioid agents cause adverse cardiovascular effects in dogs, including bradycardia and histamine-mediated hypotension (Lumb and Jones, 1984). Anticholinergic agents can be administered to prevent or treat opioid-induced bradycardia. The mixed agonist/antagonist, butorphanol, is a useful agent for premedicating dogs with respiratory disorders since it has been shown to produce only minimal changes in cardiopulmonary function (Trim, 1983).

Neuroleptanalgesic mixtures (droperidol/fentanyl, acepromazine/pethidine, acepromazine/etorphine) can be used with reasonable safety in dogs with mild to moderate respiratory insufficiency and may be the safest agents for controlling dogs which are frantic as a result of severe extrapulmonary obstructive disease. These drug combinations, which can be administered intravenously or intramuscularly, are probably best employed at a low dose rate in this situation. The synergistic effect of the two agents produces more profound sedation or narcosis than is possible using the same dosage of either agent alone. This permits effective sedation at a lower dose rate and helps to minimize adverse side effects. Oxygen should probably be administered by a face mask as the drugs take effect. The same precautions and contraindications apply to the use of such mixtures as when the agents are administered independently.

Anticholinergic agents, such as atropine and glycopyrronium

(glycopyrrolate), are useful in many forms of obstructive respiratory disorders, both to reduce salivation and prevent excessive secretion from glands of the tracheobronchial tree. These agents have the added advantage of permitting some bronchodilatation as a result of their vagolytic action. The only contraindication is in patients where the tracheobronchial secretions are already thick and viscid or purulent. In these patients, an increase in viscosity of the secretions would be detrimental.

INDUCTION

Preoxygenation is a useful adjunct to anaesthetic induction in any debilitated animal and is particularly valuable in patients with respiratory disease. The technique of preoxygenation involves allowing the patient to breathe 100% oxygen by face mask for 5 min prior to induction to ensure maximim tissue saturation. Prior to, or during, preoxygenation an intravenous catheter should be introduced into an accessible vein for the administration of an intravenous induction agent and intravenous fluids during maintenance. Gentle handling of the patient is crucial at this time to minimize excitement and to prevent unnecessary disturbance in the breathing pattern.

The actual method of anaesthetic induction is best determined in the light of the veterinarian's own individual experience but, in general, intravenous induction with a thiobarbiturate is satisfactory. This method of induction has the advantage of allowing rapid control of the airway. In keeping with the principles of good anaesthetic practice, when thiobarbiturates are used they should be administered at the minimum effective dose rate. Large doses of barbiturates cause marked respiratory depression and are ill-advised, particularly in patients with moderate to severe respiratory insufficiency. The end point of administration should be when the animal just loses consciousness and the jaw is sufficiently relaxed to allow intubation. Such a dose is sometimes referred to as a hypnotic or 'sleep' dose. One potential advantage of thiobarbiturates in obstructive pulmonary disease is that these agents have been shown to spare mucociliary clearance in the canine lung both during and after anaesthesia (Forbes and Gamsu, 1979).

Induction of narcosis using an opioid such as oxymorphone, has been recommended for patients with respiratory disease (Aaron and Crowe, 1985). If such a technique is used, preoxygenation is imperative and the animal should be intubated as soon as possible after the onset of unconsciousness so that ventilation can be controlled if necessary. Intubation is often difficult following induction with opioid agents but can be facilitated if the larynx is desensitized with a local anaesthetic spray. Opioid drugs are readily reversible with a specific antagonist, such as naloxone, should this become necessary.

In cats, ketamine can be used for intravenous induction of anaesthesia. It may even be the agent of choice when potentially reversible obstructive airway disease is present as ketamine relaxes bronchial smooth muscle and reduces airway resistance (Hirshman *et al.*, 1979; White, Way and Trevor, 1982). Salivation can be profuse following the administration of ketamine, so premedication with atropine or glycopyrronium is advisable.

In highly excitable or stressed animals, rapid induction of anaesthesia with an intravenous agent may be the only safe and expeditious method, although induction with an inhalational agent can sometimes be performed effectively. Inhalational induction using a face mask has much to recommend it in cases of upper airway obstruction (Lowe, 1986). Alternatively, small dogs and cats may be anaesthetized with volatile agents in a purpose-built induction chamber. Animals with a tracheostomy are best anaesthetized by delivering anaesthetic vapour directly through the tracheostomy tube. With this technique, there is often negligible resistance from the patient, probably because the olfactory structures are bypassed.

All patients should be intubated with a cuffed endotracheal tube as soon as possible following induction. This not only ensures protection of the airway but also facilitates intermittent positive pressure ventilation (IPPV) of the lungs, if necessary. The endotracheal tube should be inserted to the mid-tracheal region and should be firmly secured with tape or gauze bandage. An oxyscope —essentially, a laryngoscope with an oxygen line attached—can help to prevent cyanosis while facilitating intubation. Intermittent suctioning of the endotracheal tube may be necessary in cases of obstructive respiratory disease where mucus plugging could occur.

Where there is unilateral ventilatory impairment it is crucial to ensure that the 'good' side is positioned uppermost immediately after the induction of anaesthesia and intubation. Unilateral ventilatory impairment may result from conditions such as pulmonary contusion or diaphragmatic hernia. A fatality was reported following induction of anaesthesia in a cat with diaphragmatic hernia, when the affected side was inadvertently positioned uppermost (Garson, Dodman and Baker, 1980).

MAINTENANCE

Maintenance techniques may involve either allowing the patient to breathe spontaneously or the implementation of controlled ventilation. Spontaneous breathing techniques are adequate when respiratory insufficiency is mild, but in other cases it is advisable to institute IPPV. Intermittent positive pressure ventilation is an essential part of maximal support techniques. Ventilation of the lungs can be performed manually or mechanically. Manual ventilation is silent and, in experienced hands, may provide useful information about the distensibility (compliance) of the lungs. Mechanical ventilation is, however, much more convenient since it allows the anaesthetist freedom for other activities, but its use presupposes the availability of an anaesthetic ventilator.

Inhalational agents should be used to maintain unconsciousness in all but the shortest anaesthetic procedures. The choice of agent is probably less important than the way in which it is employed. Halothane or isoflurane are probably the best agents to select in most instances. Both of these agents are particularly useful when there is bronchospastic disease as they prevent allergic and non-allergic bronchoconstriction (Hirshman, 1981). The inspired concentration of the volatile agent should be the minimum that is compatible with the surgery being performed. This is the concentration which just prevents movement in response to painful stimulation while providing adequate muscle relaxation to facilitate the surgery. When IPPV is used, more efficient alveolar ventilation may permit a slightly lower inspired anaesthetic concentration to be used than would be necessary with a spontaneous breathing technique.

Sometimes, nitrous oxide may be used to supplement the more potent volatile anaesthetic in order to reduce the dose requirement of the latter. For example, the inspired halothane concentration may be reduced by 22% when nitrous oxide is employed (DeYoung and Sawyer, 1980). Nitrous oxide should not be used when there is a pneumothorax since it will diffuse into the intrapleural gas pocket and cause it to expand. It has been shown experimentally in dogs that a pneumothorax can double in size in 10 min when 75–80% nitrous oxide is respired (Saidman and Eger, 1965). If nitrous oxide is used, care should be taken to ensure that the inspired fraction of oxygen is sufficient to maintain appropriate blood and tissue oxygen tensions. When there is any doubt about the ability of the patient to maintain normal oxygen levels, it is probably best to avoid nitrous oxide.

The use of neuromuscular blocking drugs, such as pancuronium, atracurium and vecuronium, can permit a further reduction in the inspired concentration of the volatile anaesthetic agent by supplying muscle relaxation independently of narcosis and by suppressing reflex somatic responses to surgery. When using such a technique—a form of balanced anaesthesia—great care must be taken to ensure that unconsciousness prevails. This can be accomplished by paying careful attention to the heart rate and blood pressure to ensure that they remain stable and by looking for signs of lightening anaesthesia, such as lacrimation and salivation. Reflex contractions of limb and facial muscle, which can occur even when full doses of relaxants have been given, also indicate that the animal is awakening (Hall and Clarke, 1983).

Supportive therapy

Fluids. The intravenous infusion of a balanced polyionic electrolyte solution is beneficial for most surgical patients to compensate for water deprivation and increased fluid loss associated with surgery. An infusion rate of 2–10 ml kg^{-1} h^{-1} is usually sufficient unless extraordinary losses are incurred. The same considerations apply to patients with respiratory insufficiency although care should be taken in cases of pulmonary oedema, when over-zealous fluid therapy can aggravate the condition.

Heat. Temperature homeostasis is important for patients with respiratory disease, since hypothermia may result in shivering and an associated increase in oxygen consumption in the recovery period (Bay and Nunn, 1967). Postoperative hypoxaemia is more likely under these circumstances. Hypothermia can be minimized by a warm operating room environment, preventing draughts, warming intravenous fluids and insulating the patient from cold conductive surfaces (Waterman, 1975). Electric heating pads may be useful in some patients, but in a recent controlled clinical study, recirculating warm water pads were shown to be ineffective (Hubbell and Muir, 1985).

Humidification of the inspired gases. This aspect of inhalational anaesthesia, a frequently neglected consideration in veterinary medicine, is of particular importance in many patients with respiratory disorders. As well as minimizing heat loss which occurs when dry anaesthetic gases are respired, humidification helps to prevent desiccation of the tracheobronchial mucosa and preserves the normal ciliary action (Berry and Hughes-Davis, 1972). Humidification of the inspired gases is particularly important when non-rebreathing anaesthetic circuits are used and has been shown in one study to reduce the incidence of postoperative pulmonary complications in dogs (Dodman and Britobabapulle, 1979).

Monitoring

Heart rate, respiratory rate and depth, colour of mucous membranes, and ocular reflexes should be monitored and recorded at

5–10 min intervals (Dodman, Seeler and Court, 1984). In spontaneously breathing patients, it is helpful to measure the MRV at intervals during anaesthesia using a respirometer to confirm that ventilation is adequate. If ventilation is inadequate, it should be controlled by IPPV. The definitive method of quantitating the efficiency of ventilation and gas exchange is arterial blood gas analysis but, unfortunately, facilities for this rarely exist in veterinary practice. Positive pressure ventilation, although generally helpful, may have serious detrimental effects on the cardiovascular system if employed over-enthusiastically (Mushin *et al.*, 1979). Accordingly, it is recommended that the inflation pressure of the lungs be monitored and kept to the minimum necessary to effect adequate ventilation (normally less than 20 cmH$_2$O). In conditions where there is loss of pulmonary compliance, higher pressures may be necessary. Under these circumstances, the cardiovascular system should be monitored closely, including serial measurements of systemic arterial blood pressure.

RECOVERY

A supervised recovery is no less important than a closely monitored anaesthetic induction or maintenance. The patient should be observed for signs of respiratory distress or evidence of postoperative pain. Supplementary oxygen is particularly indicated during this period and can be administered by the nasal or transtracheal route or by means of an oxygen cage (Court, Dodman and Seeler, 1985). Attention to fluid balance and prevention of heat loss are also important.

The alleviation of postoperative pain is a consideration which is sometimes overlooked. Apart from the humanitarian aspects, it is imperative that all patients are permitted to recover quietly and comfortably for physiological reasons. Stress and anxiety have a detrimental effect upon a patient which already has some degree of respiratory insufficiency. The pain of abdominal incisions or thoracotomy wounds can prevent normal respiratory excursions and compound existing ventilatory impairment. In these situations, opioid analgesics can improve ventilation appreciably. Alternatively, local anaesthetic techniques may be useful in specific instances. Intercostal nerve blocks with the long-acting local anaesthetic agent, bupivacaine, will control the pain of a thoracotomy incision for several hours after surgery (Berg and Orton, 1986). Techniques involving the intrathecal or epidural administration of opioid analgesics may be used more frequently in the future for postoperative analgesia (Durant and Yaksh, 1986). Whichever analgesic technique is selected it is important to strive for a peaceful and pain-free recovery.

ADDENDUM

A table listing all the specific pharmacological agents referred to in the text is provided for the convenience of the reader (Table 3). The uses, contraindications, side effects and suggested dose ranges of these agents are listed in the table.

Table 3. Indications, contraindications and side effects of drugs in respiratory disease

Agent	Indications for use in respiratory disease	Major side effects/ contraindications	Dose rate
Aminophylline	Chronic bronchitis	Cardiac dysrhythmias Excitement Incoordination	4–10 mg kg^{-1} p.o. or i.v. (dog) 2–5 mg kg^{-1} p.o. or i.v. (cat)
Terbutaline	Chronic bronchitis	—	0.1 mg kg^{-1} p.o. three times daily
Atropine	Cholinergic bronchospasm	Respiratory depression with overdose	0.02–0.4 mg kg^{-1} i.m.
Glycopyrronium (glycopyrrolate)	Cholinergic bronchospasm	—	0.01–0.02 mg kg^{-1} i.m.
Prednisolone	Feline asthma Pulmonary trauma	Hepatopathy with prolonged usage	0.25–0.5 mg kg^{-1} i.m.
Dexamethasone	Feline asthma Pulmonary trauma	Hepatopathy with prolonged usage	1–2 mg kg^{-1} i.v. or i.m.
Acepromazine	Routine premedication in patients with mild respiratory disease Calming animals whose respiratory condition is aggravated by anxiety	Respiratory depression: avoid when moderate or severe respiratory disorders are present Decreased vascular tone may cause pooling of blood and reduce cardiac output. Avoid in shock-like states	0.025–0.1 mg kg^{-1} i.m.
Morphine	Pulmonary oedema Preoperative anxiolysis and analgesia in mild respiratory disease Postoperative analgesia	Respiratory depression: avoid when respiratory disturbance is moderate/severe Histamine release Bradycardia	0.1–0.2 mg kg^{-1} i.m. (dog) 0.05–0.1 mg kg^{-1} i.m. (cat)

Table 3.   *Continued*

Agent	Indications for use in respiratory disease	Major side effects/ contraindications	Dose rate
Butorphanol	Preoperative anxiolysis and analgesia in mild respiratory disease Postoperative analgesia	Respiratory depression: avoid when respiratory disturbance is moderate/ severe	$0.1–0.4$ mg kg^{-1} i.m.
Neurolept-analgesic mixtures	Premedication of dogs with mild/moderate respiratory disorders Controlling dogs which are frantic as a result of extrapulmonary obstructive disease	Respiratory depression Bradycardia Avoid excessive doses	Depends on formulation
Thiobarbiturate	Rapid induction of anaesthesia to permit immediate control of the airway (intubation) but preoxygenate first	Respiratory depression Cardiovascular collapse in shock patients Avoid in severe cases of cardiopulmonary dysfunction	$2–10$ mg kg^{-1} i.v.
Oxymorphone	Intravenous induction of anaesthesia in struggling patients when thiobarbiturates are contraindicated (preoxygenate first and administer anticholinergic premedication)	Respiratory depression Bradycardia	$0.1–0.2$ mg kg^{-1} i.v.
Ketamine	Chemical restraint or intravenous induction in cats with respiratory disease (particularly if there is evidence of bronchoconstriction)	Prolonged recovery if too high dose rate is used	$2–5$ mg kg^{-1} i.v. ($5–10$ mg kg^{-1} i.m.)
Nitrous oxide	Supplementation of other more potent inhalational anaesthetics at induction or during maintenance of anaesthesia	Hypoxia Diffusion into gas filled spaces Contraindicated if hypoxia is present or likely to be induced. Contraindicated in pneumothorax	$50–66\%$ of the inspired mixture.
Halothane	Induction and/or maintenance of anaesthesia	Cardiac dysrhythmias	$2–4\%$ (induction) $0.5–1.5\%$ (maintenance)

Table 3. *Continued*

Agent	Indications for use in respiratory disease	Major side effects/ contraindications	Dose rate
Isoflurane	Induction and/or maintenance of anaesthesia	—	2–5% (induction) 0.5–1.5% (maintenance)
Pancuronium	Neuromuscular block	Tachycardia	0.06–0.08 mg kg^{-1} i.v.
Atracurium	Neuromuscular block	Mild histamine release	0.2–0.4 mg kg^{-1} i.v.
Vecuronium	Neuromuscular block	Contraindicated in hepatic failure	0.1–0.2 mg kg^{-1} i.v.

REFERENCES

Amis, T. C. and Kurpershoek, C. (1986). *American Journal of Veterinary Research* **47**, 2200.

Aron, D. N. and Crowe, D. T. (1985). *Veterinary Clinics of North America* **15**, 891.

Bay, J. and Nunn, J. F. (1967). *British Journal of Anaesthesia* **39**, 518.

Berg, R. J. and Orton, E. C. (1986). *American Journal of Veterinary Research* **47**, 471.

Berry, F. A. and Hughes-Davis, D. I. (1972). *Anesthesiology* **37**, 456.

Court, M. H., Dodman, N. H. and Seeler, D. C. (1985). *Veterinary Clinics of North America* **15**, 1041.

Crago, R. R., Bryan, A. C., Laws, A. K. *et al.*, (1972). *Canadian Anaesthesia Society Journal* **19**, 607.

Davis, L. E. (1979). *Journal of the American Veterinary Medical Association* **1**, 97.

DeYoung, D. J. and Sawyer, D. C. (1980). *Journal of the American Animal Hospital Association* **16**, 125.

Dodman, N. H. and Britobabapulle (1979). *Proceedings of the Association of Veterinary Anaesthetists of Great Britain and Ireland* **8**, 141.

Dodman, N. H., Seeler, D. C. and Court, M. H. (1984). *British Veterinary Journal* **140**, 505.

Durant, P. A. C. and Yaksh, (1986). *Anesthesiology* **64**, 43.

Fairley, H. B. (1981). *32nd Annual Refresher Course Lectures of the ASA (Oct.)*, 228.

Fitzpatrick, R. K. and Crowe, D. T. (1986). *Journal of the American Animal Hospital Association* **22**, 293.

Forbes, A. R. and Gamsu, G. (1979). *Anesthesiology* **50**, 26.

Frick, O. L. (1974). *41st Annual Meeting of the American Animal Hospital Association* Seminar synopsis.

Garson, H. L., Dodman, N. H. and Baker, G. J. (1980). *Journal of Small Animal Practice* **21**, 469–481.

Hall, L. W. (1971). *Wright's Veterinary Anaesthesia and Analgesia*, 7th edn, p. 147, London: Baillière Tindall.

Hall, L. W. and Clarke, K. W. (1983). *Veterinary Anaesthesia*, 8th edn. London: Baillière Tindall.

Hartsfield, S. M. (1985). *Textbook of Small Animal Surgery*, Vol. 2, 2619; ed. D. H. Slatter. Philadelphia: W. B. Saunders Co.

Haskins, S. C. (1983). *Current Veterinary Therapy*, **VIII**, 201; ed. R. W. Kirk. Philadelphia: W. B. Saunders, Co,

Hirshman, C. A. (1981). *32nd Annual Refresher Course Lectures of the ASA (Oct.)*, 111.

Hirshman, C. A., Downes, H., Farbood, A. and Bergman, N. A. (1979). *British Journal of Anaesthesia* **51**, 713.

Hubbell, J. A. E. and Muir, W. W. (1985). *Proceedings of Veterinary Midwest Anesthesia Conference* V3, Illinois.

Kotlikoff, M. I. and Gillespie, J. R. (1983). *Compendium on Continuing Education for the Practicing Veterinarian*, August, Vol. 5, **8**, 634.

Kotlikoff, M. I. and Gillespie, J. R. (1984). *Compendium on Continuing Education for the Practicing Veterinarian*, May, Vol. 6, **5**, 462.

Lowe, D. A. (1986). *37th Annual Refresher Course Lectures of the ASA (Oct)* 164.

Lumb, W. V. and Jones, E. W. (1984). *Veterinary Anesthesia*, 2nd edn, p. 176. Philadelphia: Lea & Febiger.

Marsh, H. M. (1983). *33rd Refresher Course Lectures of the ASA (Oct)*, 207.

McKiernan, B. C. (1983). *Current Veterinary Therapy*, **VIII**, 216. ed. R. W. Kirk. Philadelphia: W. B. Saunders Co.

Milledge, J. S. and Nunn, J. F. (1980). In *General Anaesthesia*, 1, 4th edn, eds. T. C. Gray, J. F. Nunn and J. E. Utting, p. 525. London: Butterworths.

Moses, B. L. and Spaulding, G. L. (1985). *Veterinary Clinics of North America*, **15**, 929.

Mushin, W. W., Rendall-Baker, L., Thompson, P. W. and Mapleson, W. W. (1979). *Automatic Ventilation of the Lungs*, 3rd edn. Oxford: Blackwell Scientific Publications.

Raffin, T. (1982). *33rd Annual Refresher Course Lectures of the ASA (Oct)*, 217.

Saidman, L. J. and Eger II. E. I. (1965). *Anesthesiology* **26**, 67.

Snyder, G. L. (1973). *Chest* **63**, 801.

Spaulding, G. L. (1987). Personal communication.

Tams, T. R. and Sherding, R. G. (1981). *Compendium on Continuing Education for the Practicing Veterinarian* Vol. 3, **11**, 986.

Tarhan, S. *et al.*, (1974). *Surgery* **74**, 720.

Tasker, J. B. (1980). *Clinical Biochemistry of Domestic Animals*, ed J. J. Kaneko. New York: Academic Press.

Trim, C. M. (1983). *American Journal of Veterinary Research* **44**, 329.

Waterman, A. (1975). *Veterinary Record* April 5, 308.

West, J. B. (1982). *Pulmonary Pathophysiology—The Essentials*, p. 171. Baltimore: Williams and Williams.

White, P. F., Way, W. L. and Trevor, A. J. (1982). *Anesthesiology* **56**, 119.

5

Anaesthesia for patients with cardiac disease

The successful management of anaesthesia in small animals with cardiac disease requires knowledge of the general health status of the patient and detailed information regarding the cardiac disease process itself. A clinical history and results of the preoperative examination will define the type and extent of any cardiovascular impairment (Schwartz, 1985). This information, together with an understanding of the physiological effects of anaesthetic agents, should enable the clinician to evaluate the anaesthetic risk.

In this review we discuss the pathophysiology of the more common cardiac disorders and the changes in technique required for the management of anaesthesia in affected patients. For a detailed discussion of the medical and surgical considerations for each disease process, the reader is referred to other texts (Edwards and Tilley, 1981; Pyle, 1983).

PATHOPHYSIOLOGY OF CARDIAC DISORDERS

Congenital cardiac disorders

Small animals with cardiac disease account for 0.5–1.0% of patients seen in clinical practice (Pyle, 1983). Ten per cent of dogs presented with clinical signs of heart disease have cardiac problems which are of congenital origin (Pyle, 1983). Congenital heart defects tend to be less prevalent in cats. In the dog the most common congenital heart defects, in descending order of prevalence, include: (1) patent ductus arteriosus; (2) pulmonic stenosis and (3) aortic stenosis. Less common congenital defects in the dog will not be discussed here but include ventricular septal defects, atrial septal defects and tetralogy of Fallot. In the cat, patent ductus arteriosus, aortic stenosis and ventricular septal defects are common while pulmonic stenosis is rare.

Patent ductus arteriosus. Phylogenically, the ductus arteriosus is the embryonic left sixth aortic arch. If the ductus arteriosus does not close after birth, shunting of blood occurs (Edwards and Tilley, 1981). Left to right shunts are the most common and are readily diagnosed. Right to left shunts tend to be diagnosed later when the owner notices exercise intolerance (Pyle, 1983).

The significance of the shunt in altering haemodynamic parameters depends on the cross-sectional area of the patent ductus. In left to right shunts, pulmonary blood flow is augmented, resulting in pulmonary hyperfusion, hypertension and congestion while systemic circulation is reduced (Weirich, Blevins and Rebar, 1978; Allen, 1982). The alterations in pulmonary haemodynamics result in an elevation in left atrial and left ventricular filling pressures and medial hypertrophy with intimal proliferation of the pulmonary artery (Weirich, Blevins and Rebar, 1978). The increase in right ventricular afterload can lead to right ventricular enlargement and increased right-sided end diastolic pressures.

Plasma aldosterone and antidiuretic hormone levels increase as the result of systemic hypotension causing a retention of fluid and an increase in venous return. The improvement in venous return and subsequent elevation of left ventricular filling pressure leads to an increase in stroke volume and subsequently, cardiac output. Over time, the left ventricle enlarges and hypertrophies in order to maintain adequate cardiac output and systemic circulation. Ventricular dilatation could eventually lead to mitral insufficiency due to stretching of the atrioventricular valvular annulus. Rises in left ventricular work and myocardial oxygen demand are traceable to the compensatory mechanisms of augmented stroke volume and myocardial hypertrophy.

In general, if systemic blood flow is normal, the kinetics of inhalant anaesthetic agents are not altered (Schwartz, 1985). The patient with a patent ductus arteriosus tolerates haemodynamic changes associated with positive pressure ventilation because of the increased pulmonary blood flow which exists in such patients (Stoelting and Miller, 1984). Heart rate should not be altered preoperatively by administration of anticholinergics. The increased heart rate associated with the use of an anticholinergic does not allow adequate ventricular filling, and increases myocardial work and oxygen demand. After ligation of the ductus, a reflex reduction in heart rate following the increase in systemic pressure is to be expected. Moderate decreases in heart rate are not clinically significant and seldom require treatment, since the bradycardia is usually self-limiting. If, however, the decrease in heart rate is significant, then administration of an anticholinergic such as atropine is indicated. Moderate intraoperative reductions in peripheral vascular resistance due to anaesthetic agents are tolerated and may reduce the magnitude of a left to right shunt prior to ligation.

Pulmonic stenosis. Recently, the clinical, diagnostic and prognostic data from 29 cases of pulmonic stenosis were reported (Fingland, Bonagura and Myer, 1986). Surgical correction of the defect is necessary to prevent heart failure when the patient shows clinical signs of heart disease or if the pressure gradient between peak pulmonary systolic and peak right ventricular systolic pressures exceeds 70 mmHg.

The increased resistance to outflow due to stenosis of the right ventricular outflow tract causes a pressure drop across the stenotic region. Magnitude of the pressure gradient is dependent upon four factors: (1) resistance to outflow; (2) presence or absence of tricuspid regurgitation; (3) velocity and turbulence of blood flow; and (4) the inotropic state of the right ventricle (Fingland, Bonagura and Myer, 1986). Pulmonary arterial pressures and pulmonary perfusion may be normal or reduced. In order to maintain adequate cardiac output, peak right ventricular systolic pressure must increase. Elevation of central venous pressure and right ventricular filling pressures secondary to tricuspid insufficiency may lead to dilatation of the right ventricle and an increased stroke volume. An increase in the right ventricular inotropic state also increases systolic pressures in the right ventricle. Over the long term, right ventricular hypertrophy develops and eventually, in severe cases, decompensation and failure of the right side can occur.

Blood flow is dependent upon the pressure gradient across the obstructed region of the right ventricular outflow tract. During anaesthesia, heart rate should be maintained or allowed to decrease slightly to allow for adequate filling of the right ventricle. Central venous pressure and venous return should be maintained so that there is an adequate preload. Anaesthetic agents with minimal myocardial depressant activities should be used.

Aortic stenosis. Aortic stenosis results in a reduction in size of the left ventricular outflow tract and an elevated resistance to blood flow. Subvalvular lesions tend to be more common in dogs while supravalvular lesions are seen more often in cats (Edwards and Tilley, 1981; Pyle, 1983). If the pressure gradient across the stenotic region is greater than 80 mmHg, the stenosis is considered severe (Edwards and Tilley, 1981).

In order to compensate for increased resistance in the outflow tract, there is left ventricular hypertrophy and an enhanced inotropic state of the left ventricle. This sequence of events elevates myocardial work and oxygen demand. If myocardial oxygen demand exceeds oxygen supply, dysrhythmias or left ventricular failure may occur.

Surgical correction of aortic stenosis is not practical in clinical practice at this time, as cardiac bypass equipment is required. Recent reports suggest that cardiac bypass techniques may be feasible in small animal referral institutions (Klement *et al.*, 1987). However, dogs or cats with this congenital defect may need to be anaesthetized for other purposes. In patients with aortic stenosis, hypertension and significant reductions in venous return are poorly tolerated. Intraoperatively, heart rate should be maintained near or below normal values in order for the left ventricle to maintain an adequate filling time. Major or prolonged changes in either rate or rhythm can result in substantial reductions in left ventricular efficiency. High aortic pressures result in a substantial reduction in cardiac output in a patient with aortic stenosis. Excessive cardiac depression due to anaesthetics is associated with substantial reductions in systemic pressure and coronary blood flow. Systemic pressure is best controlled with pharmacological agents which act on the peripheral vasculature and not on the heart.

Acquired disorders of the heart

Mitral insufficiency. Chronic mitral valvular disease often leads to mitral insufficiency and is a frequent cause of congestive heart failure in the older dog (Ettinger, 1983; Kittleson *et al.*, 1984), Mitral insufficiency is most commonly seen in small to medium size breeds. In the larger breeds of dog, mitral insufficiency often occurs secondary to myocardial disease. Pathologically, changes may be seen in mitral valves of susceptible dogs at 2–3 years of age, while clinical signs are often not present until 8 or 9 years of age.

Severe cases of mitral insufficiency, with a major impact on haemodynamics, are more likely to be seen in the older dog. Dogs with mitral valvular regurgitation in which mean left atrial pressure exceeds 30 mmHg may develop significant cardiopulmonary disease (Miller *et al.*, 1986). Under these circumstances, myocardial work and oxygen demand are often substantially increased. In the early stages of the disease, gradual atrial enlargement is associated with mitral regurgitation. Left atrial pressure becomes elevated leading to left ventricular overload and dilatation. Stroke volume increases but the ejection fraction is reduced due to regurgitant flow. Ventricular hypertrophy occurs due to the increased workload. There is a gradual elevation in pulmonary venous pressure and pulmonary congestion develops. This results in increased work of breathing, decreased compliance, potential $\dot{V}/\dot{Q}$ abnormalities, and in extreme situations, hypoxaemia. If the condition is sufficiently severe, right heart failure may also occur as a sequela.

When mitral insufficiency is advanced, the anaesthetist should attempt to maintain cardiac output by ensuring that heart rate is normal or is only slightly elevated. It is equally important to minimize any anaesthetic-related inotropic depression of the myocardium (Arens, 1985). Peripheral vascular resistance should be reduced to improve forward flow and to reduce the degree of mitral regurgitation. In this respect, the use of nitrous oxide should be discouraged as it increases peripheral vascular resistance (Table 1). To ensure that cardiac output is maintained normal central venous pressure should be preserved through administration of fluids. In instances where pulmonary complications are evident, intermittent positive pressure ventilation (IPPV) of the patient is of value.

Ventricular hypertrophy and cardiomyopathy. Hypertrophy of either ventricle results in a decrease in diastolic compliance, ventricular filling and stroke volume. A reduction in left ventricular compliance may result from hypertrophic changes of the myocardium secondary to aortic stenosis, mitral regurgitation or cardiomyopathy. Reductions in right ventricular compliance occur in association with cor pulmonale or pulmonic stenosis.

In all forms of cardiomyopathy, the inotropic state of the ventricles is diminished. In the dog, both the dilated and hypertrophic forms of cardiomyopathy have been reported (Liu, Maron and Tilley, 1979); Thomas *et al.*, 1984; Gooding, Robinson and Mews, 1986). In the cat, dilated, hypertrophic and restricted forms of cardiomyopathy have been reported, either as primary conditions or secondary to other diseases (Tilley, 1981; Liu, Peterson and Fox, 1984; Moise and Dietze, 1986; Moise *et al.*, 1986).

Canine hypertrophic cardiomyopathy is idiopathic, and similar in nature to the disease which occurs in cats and man. Hypertrophic cardiomyopathy in the dog can be associated with a variable subaortic pressure gradient which is haemodynamically similar to a dynamic, muscular subaortic stenosis (Thomas *et al.*, 1984). The left ventricle is often small in volume and hyperdynamic, and systolic mitral regurgitation can occur. Clinically, elevated heart rates in the perioperative period can result in an increase in the obstructive pressure gradient with a subsequent reduction in aortic pulse pressure and coronary perfusion. Similarly, any anaesthetic procedure which results in a diminished left ventricular diastolic volume, a diminished ventricular afterload or an increased inotropic state may cause a reduction in cardiac output and systemic pressure (Thomas *et al.*, 1984).

Table 1. Effects of anaesthetic drugs on determinants of cardiac function*

	A. Direct effects		
Preload	Contractility	Afterload	Heart rate
↓	↓	↓	↓
	B. Indirect effects†		

Preload

Increased	Decreased	Unchanged
1. Barbiturates	1. Butyrophenones	1. Belladonna derivatives
2. Inhalation anaesthetics	2. Phenothiazines	2. Dissociative agents
	3. Narcotics	3. Nitrous oxide
	4. Benzodiazepines	4. Muscle relaxants
	5. Xylazine	

Contractility

Increased	Decreased	Unchanged
1. Dissociative agents	1. Butyrophenones	1. Belladonna derivatives
2. Morphine (low doses)	2. Phenothiazines	2. Benzodiazepines
	3. Narcotics	3. Xylazine
	4. Barbiturates	4. Phenothiazines (?)
	5. Inhalation anaesthetics	5. Muscle relaxants
	6. Nitrous oxide	

Afterload

Increased	Decreased	Unchanged
1. Dissociative agents	1. Butyrophenones	1. Belladonna derivatives
2. Nitrous oxide	2. Phenothiazines	2. Muscle relaxants
	3. Narcotics	
	4. Benzodiazepines	
	5. Xylazine	
	6. Barbiturates	
	7. Inhalation anaesthetics	

Heart rate

Increased	Decreased	Unchanged
1. Belladonna derivatives	1. Narcotics	1. Benzodiazepines
2. Butyrophenones	2. Xylazine	2. Muscle relaxants (?)
3. Phenothiazines		
4. Barbiturates		
5. Dissociative agents		
6. Nitrous oxide		
7. Inhalation anaesthetics		

↓ = Depressant effect.

† Indirect effects are modulated primarily by the amount of autonomic nervous system activity.

* Reproduced with permission from Muir, W. W. (1977). Anesthesia and the heart. *Journal of the American Veterinary Medical Association* **171**, 92.

In the cat, cardiomyopathy may be primary or secondary in nature. Cardiomyopathy of the hypertrophic or dilated form secondary to hyperthyroidism is frequently seen in clinical practice (Liu, Peterson and Fox, 1984; Moise and Dietze, 1986; Moise *et al.*, 1986). Cardiac enlargement is due to the effects of elevated circulating thyroxine (T_4) levels, with an increased myocardial workload. Hyperthyroidism with cardiomegaly results in increases in dp/dt, heart rate, systemic arterial pressure, cardiac index, myocardial work, myocardial oxygen demand, and a reduction in cardiac efficiency, and is often associated with secondary mitral valve incompetence (Tilley, Liu and Fox, 1983; Moise and Dietze, 1986).

Care must be taken in the preoperative period to assess adequately the severity of cardiomyopathy when present in hyperthyroid cats. Rhythm disturbances and conduction abnormalities are associated with all forms of feline cardiomyopathy.

Dilatation cardiomyopathy in cats is associated with left atrial enlargement, left ventricular dilatation and failure of the heart (Tilley, 1981; Moise *et al.*, 1986). There is increased venous pressure with slowed peripheral circulation. While pulmonary oedema is not a major clinical problem, heart failure results in pulmonary congestion, pleural effusion and low cardiac output. This form of cardiomyopathy is most often refractory to treatment.

In feline hypertrophic cardiomyopathy, reduced ventricular compliance and an increase in ventricular end diastolic pressure results in resistance to ventricular filling (Tilley, 1981). Frequently, the left atrium is dilated and pulmonary oedema may be present (Tilley, 1981; Lord *et al.*, 1974). It is uncertain whether dynamic obstruction of the left ventricular outflow tract occurs (Tilley, 1981; Tilley, Liu and Fox, 1983; Thomas *et al.*, 1984).

Restrictive feline cardiomyopathy, which is relatively uncommon, is characterized by severe endocardial fibrosis. Endocardial thickening of septal and left ventricular walls is present, most prominently in the regions of the left ventricular inflow and outflow tracts (Tilley, Liu and Fox, 1983). The fibrosis reduces left ventricular compliance and results in interference with filling of the left ventricle. Enlargement of the left atrium occurs secondary to increased left ventricular end diastolic pressure.

In anaesthetizing small animal patients with cardiomyopathy, it is of paramount importance to minimize myocardial depression and to maintain stroke volume and cardiac output by selection of appropriate anaesthetic agents. Heart rate should be maintained near or below normal rates in order to prevent the dynamic obstruction to left ventricular outflow which is associated with tachycardia. Increases in heart rate in the cat have been shown to increase end diastolic pressure and reduce ventricular performance

(Tilley, Liu and Fox, 1983). High preoperative heart rates, such as those associated with uncontrolled hyperthyroidism in cats, should be controlled with propranolol or a more specific β_1-adrenergic blocker prior to surgery (Muir and Sams, 1984). Dysrhythmias and conduction abnormalities must be controlled perioperatively and blood volume must be maintained to ensure adequate venous return. If obstruction of the left ventricular outflow tract is present, then it is necessary to: (1) increase the preload to ensure adequate filling; (2) maintain or increase afterloads and (3) reduce myocardial contractility and heart rate (Liu, Maron and Tilley, 1979; Thomas, 1985). By taking these steps the anaesthetist can reduce the effect of the restricted left ventricular outflow tract on haemodynamic performance.

Pericardial effusion and cardiac tamponade. The rate and volume of fluid accumulation in the pericardial sac determines whether pericardial effusion progresses to cardiac tamponade. As the severity of the condition progresses, there is increased interference with ventricular filling, requiring increased filling pressures to maintain cardiac output. Cardiac tamponade occurs when increased intrapericardial pressure results in cardiac compression (Wingfield, 1981). As pericardial pressure increases, ventricular filling will only occur when diastolic pressures exceed pericardial pressures (Lake, 1983). The continuing decline in the cardiac transmural pressure gradient leads to a decreased ventricular diastolic volume and stroke volume (Reed and Thomas, 1984).

With pericardial tamponade, right and left ventricular end diastolic pressures gradually increase and ultimately there is equalization of diastolic pressures throughout the heart. Left ventricular stroke volume decreases, as reduction in venous return to the left atrium is caused by right ventricular compression. Stroke volume becomes fixed, cardiac output is reduced and there is an increase in both the systemic and pulmonary venous pressures. Cardiac output becomes rate-limited. There is compensatory tachycardia, with arterial and venular vasoconstriction due to increased sympathetic nervous system activity (Lake, 1983). As central venous pressure increases, venous return becomes monophasic and occurs during ventricular systole (Wingfield, 1981). With increasing intrapericardial pressure, venous return progressively decreases leading to further reduction in cardiac output. Compensatory mechanisms are effective early in the course of the disease, but as pericardial fluid continues to accumulate, the compliance of the pericardial sac diminishes resulting in a rapid and dramatic increase in intrapericardial pressure which precipitates a life-threatening situation. Preoperative percutaneous pericardiocentesis, following use of a local analgesic such as lignocaine, should be attempted in all cases where tamponade exists. With removal of only small amounts of fluids, substantial improvement in cardiac function can be expected.

Vagal tone in these patients is enhanced (Lake, 1983). Anticholinergics should be used pre- and intraoperatively in order to prevent onset of bradycardia due to surgical manipulation of the pericardium. Bradycardia, if it occurs, results in a dramatic decrease in cardiac output. The anaesthetist should be prepared to administer agents such as dopamine or dobutamine to maintain inotropic and chronotropic functions.

When anaesthetizing a dog or cat with pericardial effusion, vascular volume must be maintained to ensure adequate venous return. In this manner, an elevated effective filling pressure will aid in the filling of the ventricles. Negative inotropic or chronotropic anaesthetic agents should be avoided. In addition, pharmacological agents which cause excessive peripheral vasodilatation or reduce venous return should also be avoided. Finally, it is best to avoid controlled ventilation in patients with cardiac tamponade prior to thoracotomy as the resultant increase in mean intrathoracic pressure while the chest is closed will impair venous return and enhance cardiac tamponade (Lake, 1983; Stoelting and Miller, 1984). When IPPV is necessary, the tidal volume should be reduced and the ventilatory rate increased to minimize the impact on cardiac function (Thomas, 1986).

ANAESTHETIC CONSIDERATIONS

General anaesthesia should provide analgesia, unconsciousness, muscle relaxation, and suppression of autonomic or somatic reflexes which result from surgical intervention. Patients with heart disease are often anaesthetized for surgical procedures involving other body systems. With these animals, it is important to be meticulous in the provision of anaesthetic care and to select the anaesthetic technique appropriate for the severity of the cardiac condition (Stoelting and Miller, 1984). Patents may be haemodynamically compensated, with or without therapy, or may be decompensated. When there is only minor impairment of cardiovascular function, good anaesthetic technique with appropriate monitoring may be all that is required. If the patient is unstable, however, then the response to general anaesthesia is often unpredictable and preoperative stabilization is necessary if at all possible. Only extreme emergencies should preclude the stabilization of these patients. If there is serious compromise of the cardiovascular system, then a blanced anaesthetic technique and careful monitoring will be required.

The clinician should be aware of the haemodynamic alterations associated with the disease process as well as the clinical pharmacology of concurrent cardiovascular medications (Jenkins and Clark, 1977; Parker and Adams, 1977; Edwards and Tilley, 1981; Tilley, 1981). Knowledge of the clinical pharmacology of the therapeutic agent(s) in question and their interactive effects with general anaesthetics is important for the successful anaesthetic management of such patients. Anaesthetic agents which exert minimal cardiovascular depression or which maintain or improve the haemodynamic state of the patient should be chosen. If, despite adequate preparation, adverse effects do occur during anaesthesia, then the clinician must remain flexible and be ready to implement alternative strategies, or terminate the procedure.

Preoperative considerations

Ancillary diagnostic aids should be utilized preoperatively, if indicated from the patient's history and the clinical examination, to confirm and quantify the extent of the cardiac disease process. Radiography, echocardiography, electrocardiographic evaluation, measurement of blood pressure and non-selective angiography provide important information in regard to the patient's health status. Results of routine laboratory tests must be evaluated carefully. Evaluation of renal function and measurement of serum electrolytes are indicated in animals with significant cardiac disease.

Premedication

Agents used in the premedication of the patient with heart disease are chosen with two important goals in mind. First, selection of the preanaesthetic agent should be aimed at reducing preoperative anxiety, or pain, or both. Adequate control of stress reduces sympathetic nervous system activity and minimizes excessive catecholamine release. Second, preanaesthetic agents should be selected to avoid further deterioration of the patient's haemodynamic status. Consideration of the cardiovascular actions of preanaesthetic agents is extremely important in patients with cardiac disease. These agents, including the anticholinergics, tranquillizers and analgesics, all have varying effects (see Table 1) on the cardiovascular system and should be selected accordingly. Drugs such as xylazine, which severely depress the cardiovascular system, should not be used.

Routine use of anticholinergic premedication has been challenged (Muir, 1977). Anticholinergics increase myocardial work, myocardial irritability and myocardial oxygen demand and thus their administration is not always desirable. The incidence of cardiac dysrhythmias and sinus tachycardia has been shown to be significantly higher prior to and after the induction of general anaesthesia in dogs which receive atropine premedication (Lumb and Jones, 1984). If anticholinergics are to be used, then careful consideration should be given to the selection of the agent. In many cardiac disorders, elevation of the heart rate is undesirable. Glycopyrronium (glycopyrrolate) may be a safer agent to use in these circumstances as it has fewer adverse cardiovascular effects than atropine when administered at recommended dosages (Lumb and Jones, 1984). In conditions in which the stroke volume is fixed and the cardiac output is rate-dependent, the use of anticholinergic agents is often indicated to prevent intraoperative bradycardia.

Phenothiazines are the most commonly used group of tranquillizers in small animal practice. Hypotension can be anticipated to follow administration of a phenothiazine as a result of α-adrenergic blockade. This may be particularly evident in patients with enhanced sympathetic nervous system activity arising from cardiac or peripheral circulatory inadequacies. On the positive side, phenothiazines protect the myocardium against adrenaline-induced ventricular dysrhythmias, reduce afterload and have useful synergistic effects with narcotic analgesics or agonist/antagonists (Lumb and Jones, 1984).

Analgesia may be provided by the administration of narcotic analgesics or one of the agonist/antagonist agents. The narcotic analgesics possess vagotonic activity and premedication with an anticholinergic agent is usually necessary. The agonist/antagonist agents such as butorphanol or nalbuphine have fewer cardiovascular side effects than the narcotic analgesics (Heel *et al.*, 1978; Sederberg *et al.*, 1981; Sawyer, Anderson and Scott, 1982; Trim, 1983; Raffe and Lipowitz, 1885) and may be safer for cardiac patients. Neuroleptanalgesic combinations such as fentanyl-droperidol (Hypnorm) or oxymorphone-diazepam may be used for premedication and may also be employed intravenously for the induction of anaesthesia.

Induction

Gentle handling is important to minimize struggling by the patient and to prevent stress at induction. A large bore venous catheter should be placed intravenously so that fluids and emergency drugs can be administered without delay. In critical cases, a central venous line should also be placed prior to induction. The central venous catheter provides the clinician with an opportunity to measure central venous pressure and offers an additional route for fluid administration.

Prior to and during induction, preoxygenation of the patient using a face mask should be performed in all patients amenable to this therapy. Only if the patient strenuously objects to the face mask should oxygenation be discontinued. Induction techniques may involve the use of injectable agents, such as the thiobarbiturates and narcotic agents, or an inhalational agent. The cardiovascular effects of the proposed induction agent (Table 1) should be evaluated with regard to the pathophysiology of the cardiac condition present (Hall and Clarke, 1983; Lumb and Jones, 1984). The thiobarbiturates permit a rapid and smooth transition to general anaesthesia and are thus convenient to use. They are, however, contraindicated in patients with severe heart disease because of their potential for severe cardiovascular depression.

The use of ketamine or injectable combinations containing ketamine in small animal patients with heart disease has been advocated (Kaplan, 1979). These recommendations should be re-examined in the light of more recent studies reporting numerous undesirable cardiovascular effects of ketamine or ketamine combinations when administered to small animals, particularly dogs (McDonell and Van Gorder, 1982; Haskins, Farver and Patz, 1985, 1986; Haskins, Patz and Farver, 1986). The use of ketamine in the small animal patient with cardiac disease is probably unwise.

Neuroleptanalgesic combinations may be used for induction of anaesthesia in cardiac patients. These drug combinations have minimal effects on cardiac contractility, cardiac output or blood pressure (Krahwinkel *et al.*, 1975), although bradycardia often occurs. Bradycardia may be prevented by prior administration of an anticholinergic such as glycopyrronium. As with all injectable agents it is important to use the lowest dose possible in order to achieve the desired effect.

Face mask inductions with an inhalational anaesthetic are recommended for patients with severely compromised cardiovascular function, unless excessive struggling or excitement is anticipated. With the advent of newer agents, such as isoflurane, inhalational induction has much to recommend it. The judicious use of nitrous oxide in combination with the volatile agent can facilitate inductions in the nervous or anxious patient.

Maintenance

Maintenance of general anaesthesia may be accomplished using either a single agent or a combination of inhalational and injectable agents. The latter technique is commonly described as a balanced anaesthetic technique (Steffey, 1983). With balanced anaesthesia, central nervous system depression and muscle relaxation can be achieved with minimal use of cardiovascular depressant agents.

Balanced techniques using inhalational agents should be considered in all severely compromised patients.

Intermittent positive pressure ventilation may be performed either manually or mechanically. The use of a mechanical ventilator, if available, is preferable. Controlled ventilation increases the complexity of the anaesthetic technique and may, if incorrectly applied, cause further deterioration in the patient's cardiovascular status. Factors which should be considered prior to, and during IPPV are described in detail elsewhere (Hall and Clarke, 1983; Lumb and Jones, 1984).

Halothane and isoflurane are examples of inhalational agents which are suitable for maintenance of anaesthesia in patients with cardiac disease. Both of these agents have a low blood gas partition coefficient. This property enables precise and rapid control over the degree of central nervous system and physiological depression which occurs (Eger, 1981; Hall and Clarke, 1983; Lumb and Jones, 1984). Methoxyflurane, with its relatively high blood gas partition coefficient, should not be used in these patients. When ventilatory function is adequate, inhalational anaesthesia with these agents is well tolerated. Halothane and isoflurane may actually be beneficial as both reduce myocardial work, mycardial oxygen demand and cardiac afterload (Table 1).

Halothane itself produces a dose-dependent depression of ventricular performance and heart rate, while moderately reducing peripheral vascular resistance (Table 1) (Eger, 1981). Depression of cardiac output is greater with halothane than with isoflurane (Eger, 1981). With halothane, in the absence of surgical stimulation, cardiac output returns to near normal because of a secondary sympathetic mediated increase in stroke volume and heart rate (Goudsouzian and Karamanian, 1984; Lumb and Jones, 1984). One serious disadvantage to the use of halothane is that it does sensitize the myocardium to the effects of circulating catecholamines and reduces the fibrillatory threshold. This is an important consideration in patients with the potential for dysrhythmias (Lumb and Jones, 1984), and may be a contraindication in certain disease states such as hyperthyroidism, phaeochromocytoma or traumatic myocarditis.

Isoflurane, when administered at a clinically useful concentration, has minimal effect on ventricular performance or cardiac output. It does, however, reduce peripheral resistance and systemic blood pressure to a greater extent than halothane (Eger, 1981; Lumb and Jones, 1984). Isoflurane has one great advantage over halothane in that it does not sensitize the myocardium to the effects of circulating catecholamines.

Nitrous oxide may be combined with either of the previously mentioned inhalational agents to reduce the required dose of the volatile anaesthetic agent. In this way, physiological depression of the cardiopulmonary system can be minimized (DeYoung and Sawyer, 1980; Hall and Clarke, 1983; Lumb and Jones, 1984). When nitrous oxide is used, care must be taken to ensure that the inspired oxygen concentration is adequate and that oxygen flux to the peripheral tissues is preserved. If the fresh gas flow of oxygen delivered to the anaesthetic circuit is inadequate, hypoxaemia will eventually result (Dohoo, McDonell and Dohoo, 1982; Haskins and Knapp, 1982). The cardiovascular effects of nitrous oxide in the healthy patient are minimal; however, under some circumstances it may exert a negative inotropic action, increase total peripheral resistance and increase heart rate (Table 1) (Muir, 1977; Booth, 1982).

The choice of muscle relaxant is based on its haemodynamic effects, reversibility and the familiarity of the clinician with a particular agent. The overall cardiovascular effects of the muscle relaxants are listed in Table 1. Vecuronium and atracurium have minimal effects on the cardiovascular system (Marshall *et al.*, 1980; Hughes and Chapple, 1981; Hall and Clarke, 1983; Jones, 1985a) Hypotension can occur after administration of high doses of atracurium. Neither agent is cumulative and both are readily reversed. Gallamine has no direct myocardial effect, but it may cause the heart rate to increase up to 20% as a result of its vagolytic activity (Lumb and Jones, 1984). A transient decrease in blood pressure is occasionally seen in the cat. Pancuronium has similar, but less severe effects on the cardiovascular system. Increases in heart rate can occur with large doses but more often changes in heart rate, cardiac output, or blood pressure are clinically insignificant (Hall and Clarke, 1983; Lumb and Jones, 1984). The duration and degree of neuromuscular blockade can be monitored with a nerve stimulator using both the train of four and tetanic stimulation (Ali and Savarese, 1976; Donati, Bevan and Bevan, 1984). All non-depolarizing agents can be reversed with cholinesterase inhibitors such as neostigmine or edrophonium. As these agents inhibit acetylcholinesterase, all three antagonists exert vagotonic activity. The bradycardia which would otherwise result can be prevented by administration of an anticholinergic agent. The reader is referred to a number of excellent reviews for a more detailed account of the pharmacology and clinical use of anticholinesterase compounds (Hall and Clarke, 1983; Lumb and Jones, 1984; Miller *et al.*, 1984; Bencini *et al.*, 1985; Jones, 1985a, b).

Maintenance techniques based on the use of narcotic analgesics have been advocated for balanced anaesthetic procedures in critical cases. The clinical application of such techniques is limited at the present time (Klide, 1985).

Monitoring

Vigilance and the timely institution of corrective measures are fundamental to successful management of anaesthesia for cardiac patients. The frequency at which clinical parameters are recorded is important. It has been recommended that vital signs be observed and recorded more frequently than the rate at which the most critical parameter changes significantly (Gavenstein and Paulus, 1982). This will prevent the anaesthetist from missing critical changes in the patient's parameters. In addition to routine monitoring (Dodman, Seeler and Court, 1984), consideration should be given to the measurement of blood pressure, central venous pressure (CVP), urinary output, ventilatory parameters, core body temperature and arterial or venous blood gases.

Measurement of blood pressure provides important information regarding organ perfusion. Peripheral vascular resistance and tissue perfusion are difficult to evaluate clinically. However, reference to the colour of the mucous membranes and capillary refill time does provide some indication of peripheral vascular tone. Direct blood pressure measurement is the most accurate, but cost and technical problems associated with its implementation (Gravenstein and Paulus, 1982) preclude its use in general practice. Even the use of a relatively simple home-made device such as the aneroid manometer (Hall and Clarke, 1983) is not as simple as it may appear. Inexpensive, accurate and easily used indirect blood pressure monitors employing the oscillometric technique are now available (Hamlin *et al.*, 1982; Coulter and Keith, 1984; Chalifoux *et al.*, 1985). If a blood pressure unit is not available, monitoring urinary output will provide indirect evidence that systemic blood pressure is adequate. Urine output will fall below 1.0 ml kg^{-1} h^{-1} if the mean systemic arterial pressure decreases below 60 mmHg.

Central venous pressure measurement provides the clinician with an additional index of cardiovascular function. Dynamic changes in CVP are often of great value in monitoring the patient with cardiac disease. Normally the CVP ranges from -2.0 cmH$_2$O to $+10$ cmH$_2$O. A steady increase in the CVP over time is indicative of cardiac failure, fluid overload or venoconstriction. The simultaneous measurement of arterial blood pressure and CVP will help the clinician determine which of these is occurring. A CVP reading above $+15$ cmH$_2$O is indicative of severe cardiovascular compromise or cardiac overload. The CVP will fall as the result of venodilatation or hypovolaemia.

Adequacy of pulmonary ventilation can be monitored using a respirometer or by arterial blood gas analysis. Excessive ventilatory depression or hypoxaemia, or both, must be avoided in patients with cardiac disease. The diseased heart is less capable of compensating for hypoxaemic episodes and is more sensitive to alterations in the balance between oxygen delivery and utilization. Hypoxaemic episodes should be prevented by ensuring an adequate level of inspired oxygen and by maintaining adequate cardiac output. Hypoxaemia (Pao_2 <60 mmHg) causes an increase in cardiac work and myocardial oxygen demand. The increase in cardiac work which results from hypoxaemia occurs primarily through a positive inotropic effect as opposed to a positive chronotropic effect (Tucker, Grover & Reeves, 1984). Substantial intraoperative blood loss should be replaced to avoid a significant reduction in the oxygen-carrying capacity of blood. Postoperative shivering, resulting from hypothermia, dramatically increases whole body oxygen consumption and increases the incidence of perioperative dysrhythmias (Zenoble and Hill, 1979; Raffe and Martin, 1983; Smith, 1985). Hypothermia should be avoided by minimizing intraoperative heat loss.

The acid–base status should be closely monitored in small animals with cardiovascular compromise. Although the sympathetic nervous system may initially accommodate for the myocardial depressant effects of acidaemia, cardiovascular depression will eventually occur (Haskins, 1977). As plasma pH decreases below 7.2 there will be moderate myocardial depression. When the pH drops below 7.1 the ability of the myocardium to respond to cardioactive agents is depressed (Haskins, 1977; Brobst, 1983). Acidaemia may also lead to venoconstriction and displacement of blood into the central circulation. This could lead to cardiac overload in patients with heart disease (Brobst, 1983). If severe alkalaemia develops, myocardial work and myocardial oxygen demand increase (Brobst, 1983).

Venous blood gas samples, collected from a jugular catheter will provide some information about cardiovascular function and blood flow in peripheral tissues. A reduction in cardiac output, mean systemic pressures of less than 60 mmHg and peripheral vasoconstriction all reduce peripheral blood flow. This causes an increase in oxygen extraction from the blood (Nunn, 1977). As a result, mean venous oxygen tension will be reduced. If the mixed venous oxygen tension is less than 30 mmHg, tissue hypoxia and possibly myocardial hypoxia could occur.

Recovery

Monitoring and supportive therapy of the cardiac patient must be continued into the recovery period. Core body temperature should be monitored. Hypothermia should be corrected when identified. Shivering can increase whole body oxygen requirement 400%

(Anderson, 1977). Oxygen supplementation is highly recommended during the period when the patient is attempting to re-establish a normothermic state. Other conditions which may necessitate postoperative oxygen supplementation include pulmonary atelectasis, fever, sepsis and pain. Postoperative oxygen therapy is indicated for the majority of cardiac patients throughout the recovery period. Techniques of oxygen administration have been described elsewhere (Court, Dodman and Seeler, 1985). Adequate control of postoperative pain by the judicious use of systemic or local analgesic agents is indicated in all patients recovering from anaesthesia (Penny and White, 1978; Taylor and Houlton, 1984).

REFERENCES

Ali, H. H. and Savarese, J. J. (1976). *Anesthesiology* **45**, 216.

Allen, D. G. (1982). *Canadian Veterinary Journal* **23**, 22.

Anderson, B. E. (1977). In *Duke's Physiology of Domestic Animals*, 8th edn, p. 1119. Ithaca: Cornell University Press.

Arens, J. F. (1985). In *Annual Refresher Course Lectures*, p. 145. Chicago: American Society of Anesthesiologists.

Bencini, A. F., Scaf, A. H. J., Agoston, S., Houwertjes, M. C. and Kersten, U. W. (1985). *British Journal of Anaesthesia* **57**, 782.

Booth, N. H. (1982). In *Veterinary Pharmacology and Therapeutics*, 5th edn, p. 175. Ames: Iowa State University Press.

Brobst, D. (1983). *Journal of the American Veterinary Medical Association* **183**, 773.

Chalifoux, A., D'Allaire, A., Blais, D., Lariviere, N. and Pelletier, N. (1985). *Canadian Journal of Comparative Medicine* **49**, 419.

Coulter, D. B. and Keith, J. C. (1984). *Journal of the American Veterinary Medical Association* **184**, 1375.

Court, M. H., Dodman, N. H. and Seeler, D. C. (1985). *Veterinary Clinics of North America* **15**, 1041.

DeYoung, D. J. and Sawyer, D. C. (1980). *Journal of the American Animal Hospital Association* **16**, 125.

Dodman, N. H., Seeler, D. C. and Court, M. H. (1984). *British Veterinary Journal* **140**, 505.

Dohoo, S. E., McDonell, W. N. and Dohoo, I. R. (1982). *Journal of the American Animal Hospital Association* **18**, 900.

Donati, F., Bevan, J. C. and Bevan, D. R. (1984). *Canadian Anaesthetist Society Journal* **31**, 324.

Edwards, N. J. and Tilley, L. P. (1981). In *Pathophysiology in Small Animal Surgery*, p. 155. Philadelphia: Lea and Febiger.

Eger, E. I. (1981). In *Isoflurane (Forane): A Compendium and Reference*, Madison: Airco.

Ettinger, S. J. (1983). In *Textbook of Veterinary Internal Medicine*, 2nd edn, p. 959. Philadelphia: W. B. Saunders.

Fingland, R. B., Bonagura, J. D. and Myer, C. W. (1986). *Journal of the American Veterinary Medical Association* **189**, 218.

Gooding, J. P., Robinson, W. F. and Mews, G. C. (1986). *American Journal of Veterinary Research* **47**, 1978.

Goudsouzian, N. and Karamanian, A. (1984). In *Physiology for the Anesthesiologist*, 2nd edn, p. 47. Norwalk: Appleton-Century-Crofts.

Gravenstein, J. S. and Paulus, D. A. (1982). In *Monitoring Practice in Clinical Anesthesia*, Philadelphia: J. B. Lippincott.

Hall, L. W. and Clarke, K. W. (1983). *Veterinary Anaesthesia*, 8th edn. London: Baillière Tindall.

Hamlin, R. L., Kittleson, M. D., Rice, D., Knowlen, G. and Seyffert, R. (1982). *American Journal of Veterinary Research* **43**, 1271.

Haskins, S. C. (1977). *Journal of the American Veterinary Medical Association* **170**, 423.

Haskins, S. C. and Knapp, R. G. (1982). *Journal of the American Veterinary Medical Association* **180**, 735.

Haskins, S. C., Farver, T. B. and Patz, J. D. (1985). *American Journal of Veterinary Research* **46**, 1855.

Haskins, S. C., Farver, T. B. and Patz, J. D. (1986). *American Journal of Veterinary Research* **47**, 795.

Haskins, S. C., Patz, J. D. and Farver, T. B. (1986). *American Journal of Veterinary Research* **47**, 636.

Heel, R. C., Brogden, R. N., Speight, T. M. and Avery, G. S. (1978). *Drugs* **16**, 473.

Hughes, R. and Chapple, D. J. (1981). *British Journal of Anaesthesia* **53**, 31.

Jenkins, W. L. and Clark, D. R. (1977). *Journal of the American Veterinary Medical Association* **171**, 85.

Jones, R. S. (1985a). *Research in Veterinary Science* **38**, 193.

Jones, R. S. (1985b). *Journal of the American Veterinary Medical Association* **187**, 281.

Kaplan, B. (1979). *Veterinary Medicine Small Animal Clinician*, 1267.

Kittleson, M. D., Eyster, G. E., Knowlen, G. G., Olivier, N. B. and Anderson, L. K. (1984). *Journal of the American Veterinary Medical Association* **184**, 455.

Klement, P., del Nido, P. J., Mickleborough, L., MacKay, C., Klement, G. and Wilson, G. J. (1987). *Journal of the American Veterinary Medical Association* **190**, 869.

Klide, A. (1985). Personal communication.

Krahwinkel, D. J., Sawyer, D. C., Eyster, G. E. and Bender, G. (1975). *American Journal of Veterinary Research* **36**, 1211.

Lake, C. (1983). *Anesthesia and Analgesia* **62**, 431.

Liu, S., Maron, B. J. and Tilley, L. P. (1979). *Journal of the American Veterinary Medical Association* **174**, 708.

Liu, S., Peterson, M. E. and Fox, P. R. (1984). *Journal of the American Veterinary Medical Association* **185**, 52.

Lord, P. F., Wood, A., Tilley, L. P. and Liu, S.-K. (1974). *Journal of the American Veterinary Medical Association* **164**, 154.

Lumb, W. V. and Jones, E. W. (1984). *Veterinary Anesthesia*, 2nd edn. Philadelphia: Lea and Febiger.

Marshall, R. J., McGrath, J. C., Miller, R. D., Docherty, J. R. and Lamar. J. C. (1980). *British Journal of Anaesthesia* **52**, 21S.

McDonell, W. W. and Van Gorder, J. (1982). In *Proceedings of the American College of Veterinary Anesthesiologists Scientific Meeting*, p. 28. Las Vegas: American College of Veterinary Anesthesiologists.

Miller, J. E., Eyster, G., DeYoung, D., Miller, B. and Robinson, N. E. (1986). *American Journal of Veterinary Research* **47**, 2498.

Miller, R. D., Rupp, S. M., Fisher, D. M., Cronnelly, R., Fahey, M. R. and Sohn, Y. J. (1984). *Anesthesiology* **61**, 444.

Moise, N. S. and Dietze, A. E. (1986). *American Journal of Veterinary Research* **47**, 1487.

Moise, N. S., Dietze, A. E., Mezza, L. E., Strickland, D., Erb, H. N. and Edwards, N. J. (1986). *American Journal of Veterinary Research* **47**, 1476.

Muir, W. W. (1977). *Journal of The American Veterinary Medical Association* **171**, 92.

Muir, W. W. and Sams, R. (1984). *Compendium of Continuing Education* **6**, 156.

Nunn, J. F. (1977). In *Applied Respiratory Physiology*, 2nd edn, p. 375. London: Butterworths.

Parker, J. L. and Adams, H. R. (1977). *Journal of the American Veterinary Medical Association* **171**, 78.

Penny, B. E. and White, R. J. (1978). *Veterinary Clinics of North America* **8**, 317.

Pyle, R. L. (1983). In *Textbook of Veterinary Internal Medicine*, 2nd edn, p. 933. Philadelphia: W. B. Saunders.

Raffe, M. R. and Lipowitz, A. J. (1985). In *Proceedings of the Second International Congress of Veterinary Anesthesia*, p. 155. Santa Barbara: Veterinary Practice Publishing Company.

Raffe, M. R. and Martin, F. B. (1983). *American Journal of Veterinary Research* **44**, 455.

Reed, J. R. and Thomas, W. P. (1984). *American Journal of Veterinary Research* **45**, 301.

Sawyer, D. C., Anderson, D. L. and Scott, J. B. (1982). In *Proceedings of the American College of Veterinary Anesthesiologists Scientific Meeting*, p. 23. Las Vegas: American College of Veterinary Anesthesiologists.

Schwartz, A. J. (1985). In *Annual Refresher Course Lectures*, p. 155. Chicago: American Society of Anesthesiologists.

Sederberg, J., Stanley, T. H., Reddy, P., Liu, W.-S., Port, D. and Gilmor, S. (1981). *Anesthesia and Analgesia* **60**, 715.

Smith, M. (1985). *Compendium on Continuing Education* **7**, 321.

Steffey, E. P. (1983). In *Animal Pain: Perception and Alleviation*, p. 133. Bethesda: American Physiological Society.

Stoelting, R. K. and Miller, R. D. (1984). In *Basics of Anesthesia*, p. 257. New York: Churchill Livingstone.

Taylor, P. M. and Houlton, J. E. (1984). *Journal of Small Animal Practice* **25**, 437.

Thomas, S. J. (1985). In *International Anesthesia Research Society Review Courses Lectures*, p. 80. Cleveland: International Anesthesia Research Society.

Thomas, S. J. (1986). In *Review Course Lectures* , p. 80. Cleveland: International Anesthesia Research Society.

Thomas, W. P., Mathewson, J. W., Suter, P. F., Reed, J. R. and Meierhenry, E. F. (1984). *Journal of the American Animal Hospital Association* **20**, 253.

Tilley, L. P. (1981). In *Pathophysiology in Small Animal Surgery*, p. 184. Philadelphia: Lea and Febiger.

Tilley, L. P., Liu, S. and Fox, P. R. (1983). In *Textbook of Veterinary Internal Medicine*, 2nd edn, p. 1029. Philadelphia: W. B. Saunders.

Trim, C. M. (1983). *American Journal of Veterinary Research* **44**, 329.

Tucker, A., Grover, R. F. & Reeves, J. T. (1984). *American Journal of Veterinary Research* **45**, 104.

Weirich, W. E., Blevins, W. E. and Rebar, A. H. (1978). *Journal of the American Animal Hospital Association* **14**, 40.

Wingfield, W. E. (1981). In *Pathophysiology in Small Animal Surgery*, p. 214. Philadelphia: Lea and Febiger.

Zenoble, R. D. and Hill, B. L. (1979). *Journal of the American Veterinary Medical Association* **175**, 840.

6

Intraoperative cardiac dysrhythmias and their management

Cardiac dysrhythmias which occur intraoperatively vary in incidence and significance. Medically, the incidence of dysrhythmias has been shown to vary with the method of monitoring. The reported frequency of dysrhythmias is low when electrocardioscopic monitoring is practised and significantly higher when a contiuously recorded ECG strip is analysed retrospectively. The significance of cardiac dysrhythmias ranges from the relatively innocuous to those which are life threatening. It should be remembered, however, that some of the less severe forms may be progressive if left untreated.

Cardiac rhythm disturbances result from changes in automaticity or from re-entry mechanisms in the conduction pathways (Wit and Rosen, 1983). Changes in automaticity can occur as the result of alterations in plasma catecholamine or electrolyte levels, changes in core body temperature, myocardial hypoxia or the administration of various anaesthetic agents. Re-entry may be caused by any of the above factors, but can also result from mechanical stretching of conduction fibres. Appropriate management of animals before and during anaesthesia will result in a significant reduction in the incidence of intraoperative dysrhythmias.

In this chapter we will examine the nature and aetiology of the various forms of cardiac rhythm disturbance which occur during anaesthesia and their treatment.

DISTURBANCES IN ATRIAL AUTOMATICITY

Supraventricular tachycardia

Supraventricular tachycardias are rapid heart rates due to a pacemaker of sinus, atrial or junctional origin (Atlee, 1980). Sinus tachycardia is the most common intraoperative dysrhythmia observed during small animal anaesthesia. A heart rate greater than 160 min^{-1} in a medium to large dog, 180 min^{-1} in a small dog, or 220 min^{-1} in a puppy or cat is classified as tachycardia (Ettinger, 1983). If the P wave has a normal configuration and position in relation to the QRS complex, then the tachycardia is sinus in origin (Fig. 1). Most abnormal P wave configurations suggest atrial tachycardia, but negative or absent P waves are associated with junctional tachycardias (Ettinger & Suter, 1970). Absence of the P wave may also suggest that the pacemaker is located below the level of the atrioventricular (AV) node and that the rhythm is ventricular in origin. In this instance, an abnormal QRS configuration would be observed (Ettinger & Suter, 1970). The term 'paroxysmal supraventricular tachycardia' refers to supraventricular tachydysrhythmias which are sudden in onset, vary in duration and end abruptly.

Heart rates which exceed two and a half times the resting value significantly interfere with cardiac output due to a decrease in ventricular filling time and subsequent reduction in stroke volume. The resting heart rate in small animals may be determined as follows: resting heart rate$=241 \times$ kg$^{-0.25}$ where 241 is a constant and kg is the body weight in kilograms to negative power 0.25 (Stahl, 1967). As the heart rate increases, myocardial oxygen demand increases, while oxygen supply remains constant or decreases. Paroxysmal tachycardia may decrease coronary circulation up to 35% (Ettinger, 1983). The lower the pacemaker is in the conduction system, the more likely it is that the dysrhythmia is haemodynamically significant (Atlee, 1980). Tachycardias originating at the AV node or lower in the conduction system may result in serious haemodynamic instability, especially in patients with pre-existing cardiac disease (Atlee, 1980).

Light planes of anaesthesia, hypotension, shock, septicaemia, hypoxia, acidosis, hyperthyroidism, hypokalaemia, primary cardiac disease and hyperthermia may all cause supraventricular tachycardia intraoperatively. Excessively high heart rates may also occur due to excitement at induction or may be the result of the administration of various pharmacological agents such as atropine (Atlee, 1980; Fox, Tilley and Liu, 1983).

In order to treat supraventricular tachycardia definitively, the underlying cause may be identified and then corrected. If the aetiology is unclear and there is an adverse effect on haemodynamic stability, a vagal manoeuvre may be attempted or appropriate doses of propranolol (Table 1) can be administered (Atlee, 1980; Fox *et al.*, 1983). An increase in vagal tone can be induced by digital pressure on the eye or over the area of bifurcation of the common carotid. If a thoracotomy or coeliotomy has been performed, direct digital pressure on the aorta may be used to decrease the heart rate to a more acceptable value. Prolonged

Table 1. Small animal emergency drug list

Indication	Drug	Concentration	Preparation	Recommended dosage*†
Atrial fibrillation	Quinidine	8% (80 mg ml⁻¹)		1.0–2.0 mg kg⁻¹ slowly
Cardiac arrest—asystole or fine fibrillation	Adrenaline	1:1000 (1.0 mg ml⁻¹)	Dilute 1 ml in 9 ml Saline (1:10 000) (0.1 mg ml⁻¹)	(0.1–0.3 mg or 1–3 ml) (0.01 mg kg⁻¹ or 0.1 ml kg⁻¹)
Anaphylaxis				
Cardiac arrest—asystole	Isoprenaline	1:5000 (0.2 mg ml⁻¹)	Dilute 1 ml in 9ml Saline (20 µg ml⁻¹)	2–10 µg kg⁻¹; 0.1–0.5 ml kg⁻¹
Cardiac stimulation Hypotension, bradycardia Prerenal failure	Dopamine	40 mg ml⁻¹	Dilute 5 ml in 1 litre D5W** to give 200 µg ml⁻¹	2–10 µg kg⁻¹ min⁻¹
Cardiac stimulation	Dobutamine	5.0%	Dilute 2 ml in 500 ml D5W** to give 200 µg ml⁻¹	1–10 µg kg⁻¹ min⁻¹
	Calcium chloride‡	10%		0.1–0.3 mEq kg⁻¹; 10 mg kg⁻¹ (1 ml 10kg⁻¹)
	Calcium gluconate§	10%		
Ventricular extrasystole Ventricular tachycardia	Lignocaine	2%		Dog: 1.0–4.0 mg kg⁻¹; 25–80 µg kg⁻¹ min⁻¹; Cat: 0.25–0.75 mg kg⁻¹; 2–6 µg kg⁻¹ min⁻¹
	Procainamide	10%		Dog; 1.0–2.0 mg kg⁻¹; 10–40 µg kg⁻¹ min⁻¹
	Propranolol¶	0.1%		40–100 µg kg⁻¹ slowly
	Methoxamine	2%		0.4 mg to 0.8 mg kg⁻¹
Hypotension	Noradrenaline	1 mg ml⁻¹	Dilute 4 ml in 500 ml D5W** (8 µg ml⁻¹)	Infuse to effect

* i.v. recommended.
† Use Soluset with Chamber (60 drops per cc).
‡ 1.36 mEq ml⁻¹.
§ 0.46 mEq ml⁻¹.
¶ Supraventricular dysrhythmias in the cat.
** 5% Dextrose solution.

bilateral carotid occlusion in man will result in cerebral ischaemia, but this does not occur in small animals. The basilar artery in the dog and cat is supplied by the vertebral arteries, which are branches of the subclavian artery.

Bradycardia

Bradycardia occurs when the sinoatrial (SA) pacemaker discharges at a slower rate than normal or when the impulses from the SA node are blocked from entering adjacent atrial myocardial muscle. If the rate is sufficiently low, escape beats occur at other sites in the atria or ventricles as new pacemakers take over. Sinus brady-cardia is the most common form of bradycardia seen intraopera-tively in small animals. Bradycardia may also be junctional in origin. A heart rate less than 80 min^{-1} in medium to large dogs or less than 110 min^{-1} in small dogs and cats under anaesthesia should be regarded as bradycardia. Sinoatrial block occurs when the SA impulse does not capture the atria, resulting in a pause in rhythm which is a multiple of the basic cycle length. Sinoatrial arrest occurs when the SA node fails to generate an impulse for a variable period of time. It may be observed in brachycephalic breeds as an incidental finding (Ettinger & Suter, 1970).

Significant reductions in heart rate to less than 60 min^{-1} may result in dramatic decreases in cardiac output and blood pressure in the dog (Muir, 1978). Halothane anaesthesia alone may cause a junctional bradycardia which can result in serious reductions in arterial blood pressure (Stoelting and Miller, 1984). Decreased myocardial oxygen supply and ventricular escape beats are poten-tial sequelae to bradycardia.

Common causes of bradycardia during the perioperative period include: anaesthetic overdose, stimulation of the parasympathetic nervous system during surgery, fluid overload, hyperkalaemia, hypothermia, renal disease or dilatative cardiomyopathy in cats (Atlee, 1980; Fox *et al.*, 1983). Premedicants such as xylazine regularly cause bradycardia preoperatively; while the use of atro-pine or acepromazine may result in bradycardia under certain circumstances (Klide, Calderwood and Soma, 1975; Muir, 1978; Tilley, 1985).

The decision as to when to treat bradycardia intraoperatively is controversial. Excessive use of anticholinergic agents periopera-tively can result in significant autonomic imbalance with the development of more severe rhythm disturbances (Muir, 1978). However, anaesthetized patients already have a reduced cardiac output and blood pressure which will become more depressed in the face of persistent bradycardia (Atlee, 1980; Tilley, 1985). Bradycardia should be treated when the heart rate continues to drop below acceptable limits. The rate at which the heart rate decreases often determines the corrective measures which must be adopted. In the non-emergency situation, time is usually available to determine and correct the primary causes of the bradycardia. In this instance the heart rate will often return to a more acceptable value before pharmacological agents are required. In situations below the lower limits of normal, the use of an anticholinergic agent such as atropine sulphate at a dose rate of 0.02 to 0.04 mg kg^{-1} i.v. is indicated.

The SA node may not respond to the administration of atropine sulphate as a result of myocardial hypoperfusion and hypoxia when the heart rate is extremely slow. In order to improve myocardial perfusion and oxygen delivery initially, a β-adrenergic agent such as isoprenaline should be administered intravenously (see Table 1). Once the heart rate increases and adequate myocardial perfusion re-established, the SA node will respond to the anticholinergic agent administered previously. Occasionally, in the hypothermic patient, the heart rate may not increase following the administration of an anticholinergic. In this situation, a decision as to whether to continue the procedure in the face of continuing bradycardia will be necessary. In our experience, bradycardias due to hypothermia do not usually respond to atropine and are not readily reversed by intraoperative rewarming techniques. In the extreme situation, the use of adrenergic agonists such as a dopamine administered as constant infusion at rates of 2.0 to 10.0 μg kg^{-1} min^{-1} may be required in order to maintain adequate cardiovascular function.

Another option for the treatment of a persistent intraoperative bradycardia is the use of a transoesophageal pacemaker (Backofen, Schauble and Rogers, 1984). While these units are not readily available in veterinary practice, their ease of application and numerous indications for use, in cardiac emergencies, warrant further investigation in veterinary medicine.

Premature atrial beats and wandering pacemakers

Atrial premature beats occasionally occur under general anaesthesia and are recognized as complexes on the electrocardioscope which appear earlier than expected in the cardiac cycle. Wandering atrial pacemakers also occur under anaesthesia and are often associated with bradycardia. A diagnostic feature of a wandering atrial pacemaker is the varying morphology of the P wave.

Treatment of atrial premature beats is not usually necessary as there are few if any haemodynamic alterations associated with these dysrhythmias. The adverse side effects of the therapeutic agents are often greater than those of the problem being treated.

Frequent premature atrial beats, or those with a multifocal origin, are potentially dangerous as they may lead to supraventricular tachycardia or atrial fibrillation (Atlee, 1980; Ettinger and Suter, 1970). Pharmacological treatment usually involves the administration of a class 1a antidysrhythmic agent such as quinidine or procainamide (see Table 1). The intravenous administration of either of these agents should be undertaken with caution as each may cause hypotension.

Atrial flutter and fibrillation

The spontaneous developmnent of atrial flutter or fibrillation during inhalational anaesthesia is rare. However, it may occur in large breeds of dogs. Atrial fibrillation is more common than atrial flutter in the canine and feline species (Ettinger and Suter, 1970). Atrial flutter is characterized electrocardiographically by rhythmic oscillations of the baseline and an AV block may be apparent (Ettinger and Suter, 1970). Atrial fibrillation is associated with a lack of defined P waves and the presence of irregular oscillations of the baseline, or f, waves (see Fig. 2). There is often a rapid, irregular ventricular rate which is sometimes associated with a pulse deficit (Ettinger, 1983). On occasion the ventricular rate may be slow.

Atrial fibrillation is frequently associated with advanced cardiac disease and may result in serious haemodynamic changes which can lead to death. Its development intraoperatively is a serious sign and every attempt should be made to determine its impact on cardiovascular function. In man, atrial fibrillation may cause cerebral blood flow to decrease by 23% of normal, while coronory and renal circulation may decrease by 40 and 20% respectively (Corday and Lang, 1974). Atrial fibrillation in the dog is commonly associated with chronic valvular disease, uni- or bilateral atrial enlargement, hypermetabolic states, hypertension and idiopathic congestive cardiomyopathy in large canine breeds (Ettinger, 1983). In cats, atrial fibrillation is primarily associated with hypertrophic cardiomyopathy (Fox *et al.*, 1983).

When a patient with atrial fibrillation is presented for surgery, the procedure should be postponed where possible and medical treatment instituted. Digoxin, propranolol and verapamil are currently recommended for this purpose (Bonagura and Muir, 1985; Johnson, 1985). Full details regarding the medical treatment of atrial fibrillation can be found elsewhere (Ettinger and Suter, 1970; Crowe and Calvert, 1984).

The development of acute atrial fibrillation intraoperatively is rare, but when it does occur, it warrants immediate evaluation. In most instances, atrial fibrillation presents as coarse fibrillation with

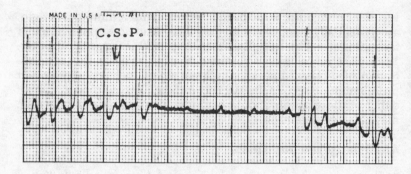

Fig. 1 Sinus tachycardia is denoted by a rapid intrinsic heart rate. The effects of carotid sinus pressure (CSP) are demonstrated.

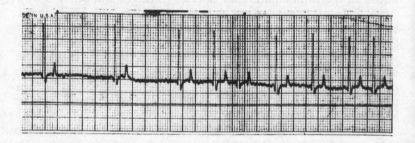

Fig. 2 Classic f waves in the baseline are seen in patients with atrial fibrillation.

a normal or slow ventricular rate. If there are no discernible haemodynamic changes, its treatment is usually unnecessary. If, however, the ventricular rate is rapid and cardiovascular stability is adversely affected, pharmacological therapy with either quinidine or propranolol is indicated in the dog. Quinidine should be administered slowly intravenously at a dose rate of 1.0 to 2.0 mg kg^{-1} (see Table 1). The anaesthetist must closely observe the animal's clinical signs during the infusion for adverse side effects such as hypotension. During the recovery period, additional quinidine may be required and should be administered at a dose rate of 6.0 to 8.0 mg kg^{-1} i.m. every 6 to 8 h, for a total of 3 doses (Bonagura and Muir, 1985).

Propranolol is indicated in the treatment of atrial fibrillation in the dog when the ventricular rate is rapid. In this situation, propranolol slows the ventricular rate by decreasing conduction through the AV node, which generally improves cardiac function by increasing diastolic filling time. In some instances, atrial fibrillation may fortuitously convert to normal sinus rhythm as a result of this treatment. In the cat, propranolol is the pharmacological agent of choice in the treatment of atrial fibrillation (see Table 1).

If there is no response to pharmacological therapy and if the ventricular rate remains high with concurrent haemodynamic instability, cardioversion should be attempted (Ettinger, 1983; Crowe and Calvert, 1984). One of our authors (N.H.D.) has successfully converted spontaneous intraoperative atrial fibrillation using neostigmine (0.02 mg kg^{-1} i.v.) in a dog.

VENTRICULAR ECTOPIC RHYTHMS

Premature ventricular contractions

Ectopic ventricular beats which occur during general anaesthesia are often related to the anaesthetic agents used, the anaesthetic technique or a light plane of anaesthesia. Premature ventricular contractions (PVCs), or extrasystoles, originate within the ventricular myocardium, or Purkinje system, and spread throughout the ventricular muscle, resulting in widened bizarre QRS complexes with T waves in the opposite direction to that of the QRS complexes (Fox *et al.*, 1983). The further away from the AV node that the ectopic pacemaker occurs, the wider and more abnormal is the QRS complex. If there is more than one abnormal complex and all are of similar configuration, this indicates that the PVCs are unifocal in origin (see Fig. 3). If the aberrant QRS complexes vary in configuration, they are multifocal in origin. An abnormal ventricular beat alternating with a normal sinus beat is referred to as bigeminy (see Fig. 4).

The coronary circulation may decrease 5% following an ectopic beat and up to 25% following frequent ventricular extrasystoles. Renal blood flow has been reported to decrease to 20% following frequent premature ventricular contractions in man (Corday and Lang, 1974). Causes of intraoperative premature ventricular contractions are numerous and include: (1) primary myocardial disease; (2) traumatic myocarditis; (3) bacterial and viral endocarditis; (4) systemic disorders; (5) physical irritants; (6) anaesthetic agents; (7) acid–base disturbances; (8) electrolyte abnormalities; (9) light plane of anaesthesia; (10) myocardial sensitization to catecholamines; and (11) hypoxaemia (Atlee, 1980; Ettinger, 1983; Fox *et al.*, 1983; Johnson, 1985).

The use of thiobarbiturates commonly results in post-intubation bigeminy of variable duration (Muir, 1977a; Musselman, 1976). Moderate increases in heart rate, blood pressure, or both, have

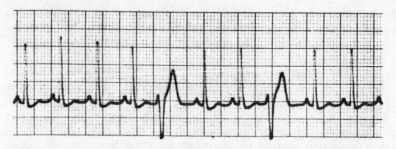

Fig. 3 Premature ventricular contractions are identified by the fact that they are premature and that the QRS complex is widened and bizarre.

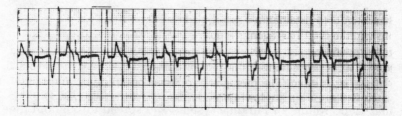

Fig. 4 Normal sinus beats alternating with premature ventricular contractions is referred to as bigeminy.

been associated with this phenomenon, which is now thought to be related to an imbalance in autonomic tone (Muir, 1977b). The incidence of thiobarbiturate-induced bigeminy is directly related to the type of thiobarbiturate used, the total dose administered, the concentration of the thiobarbiturate solution, and the rate of administration (Muir, 1977a).

Halogenated hydrocarbons, such as halothane, sensitize the myocardium to the actions of catecholamines and may result in the development of ventricular extrasystoles (Munson and Tucker, 1975; Sumikawa, Ishizaka and Suzaki, 1983; Metz and Maze, 1985). This sensitization is thought to occur primarily through postsynaptic myocardial α_1-adrenergic receptors with a lesser contribution from the β_1-adrenergic receptors in the myocardium (Maze and Smith, 1983; Spiss, Maze and Smith, 1983). The degree of sensitization of the myocardium by halothane was not found to alter over the clinically useful range of inspired halothane concentrations (Metz and Maze, 1985), but fasting and the use of xylazine or thiobarbiturates were found to increase sensitization of the myocardium by halothane (Muir, Werner and Hamlin, 1975; Atlee and Malkinson, 1980; Atlee and Flaherty, 1983).

The methyl-ethyl ethers such as methoxyflurane, enflurane or isoflurane cause minimal or no cardiac sensitization and are preferable to the alkanes, such as halothane, in this context (Joas and Stevens, 1971; Munson and Tucker, 1975). It has been suggested that the anaesthetist change from halothane to isoflurane anaesthesia in situations where ventricular extrasystoles occur as the result of halothane anaesthesia and myocardial sensitization to catecholamines (Hubbell *et al.*, 1984). This practice, however, is not without its critics (Maze and Smith, 1985).

In general, infrequent, unifocal ventricular extrasystoles are not treated medically. While they may not be haemodynamically significant, they do indicate some underlying problem which should be identified and corrected if possible. If the premature ventricular beats are multifocal in origin, or if they occur at a rate of 6 or more min^{-1}, then the underlying cause should be rapidly determined and corrected. If the underlying cause cannot be determined and corrected, the dysrhythmia should be treated pharmacologically before it progresses to a more serious disturbance with even greater haemodynamic consequences. In situations where the R wave of the ectopic ventricular beat falls on the T-wave of the preceding beat, it should be considered an ominous sign, as a ventricular tachycardia or fibrillation may result. Treatment should be instituted rapidly in this instance.

Intraoperative premature ventricular contractions in the dog may be treated with intravenous lignocaine (see Table 1). In most instances, an initial 1.0 to 2.0 mg kg^{-1} intravenous bolus of lignocaine is effective in eliminating ventricular extrasystoles in the dog (see Table 1). Occasionally, the therapeutic effects of lignocaine will wear off in 20 to 30 min. If this occurs, an additional bolus is administered and an intravenous infusion of lignocaine is started. The infusion rate is normally 25.0 to 80.0 μg kg^{-1} min^{-1} in the dog. The therapeutic plasma lignocaine level is around 6 μg ml^{-1} whilst levels above 8 μg ml^{-1} are toxic.

If lignocaine is not efficacious, then consideration should be given to the administration of procainamide. Procainamide may be administered at a dose of 1.0 to 2.0 mg kg^{-1} intravenously in the dog. This agent should be injected slowly as ganglion blockade with subsequent hypotension can occur. In those instances where the ectopic beats return after a period of time, procainamide may be administered at a constant rate of infusion of 10.0 to 40.0 μg kg^{-1} min^{-1}. The therapeutic plasma concentration for procainamide is approximately 8.0 to 16.0 μg ml^{-1}, while levels above 20 μg are toxic.

In the cat, lignocaine must be administered with caution (see Table 1). Propranolol is the pharmacological agent of choice for the treatment of intraoperative ventricular extrasystoles in this species. Procainamide should not be used in the cat.

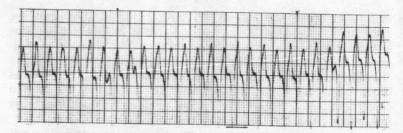

Fig. 5 Three or more premature ventricular contractions in a row is defined as ventricular tachycardia.

Ventricular tachycardia

The occurrence of three or more premature ventricular contractions in sequence is defined as ventricular tachycardia (see Fig. 5). Where a ventricular pacemaker is operating independently and is uninfluenced by atrial activity, the ventricular rhythm is termed idioventricular.

The presence of capture beats or fusion beats in the ECG tracing indicates that AV dissociation has not occurred. In this situation, if the P wave reaches the AV node when it is not refractory, the electrical impulse will be conducted throughout the myocardium. A normal P-QRS complex will appear and is referred to as a capture beat. If a P wave occurs at the same time as an ectopic ventricular beat, then a complex similar to a normal complex will occur. This is termed a fusion beat.

Frequent or multifocal ventricular extrasystoles may progress to ventricular tachycardia if the underlying cause is not corrected. Ventricular tachycardia is a serious dysrhythmia which can rapidly lead to cardiac arrest. High ventricular rates can reduce coronary perfusion by up to 40% and reduce cerebral and renal blood flow by up to 40 and 60% respectively (Corday and Lang, 1974; Atlee, 1980; Ettinger, 1983). In the dog, circulatory function rapidly deteriorates as the ventricular rate increases from 100 to 140 min^{-1} (Tilley, 1985).

Causes of ventricular tachycardia include those which result in premature ventricular extrasystoles such as re-entry. Intractable ventricular tachycardia is often associated with primary cardiac disease such as infarction.

Acute pharmacological treatment of ventricular tachycardia in the dog includes the use of lignocaine or procainamide; the techniques employed are similar to those used in the treatment of ventricular extrasystoles (see Table 1). In the cat, either quinidine or propranolol are the agents of choice. In both species, cardio-version with an externally synchronized DC non-phasic defibrillator in conjunction with lignocaine is indicated in the treatment of ventricular tachycardias which are sustained despite pharmacological therapy.

DISTURBANCES OF CONDUCTION

Atrioventricular blocks

First and second degree heart blocks can occur spontaneously intraoperatively. A first degree heart block is diagnosed when the PR interval is greater than 0.13 s in the dog and cat (see Fig. 6). The increased PR interval results from a delay in conduction through the AV node. If a P wave is intermittently not followed by a QRS complex, there is a failure of conduction through the AV node. This type of rhythm is called a second degree AV block. When the PR interval increases in duration until a QRS complex is dropped, this is referred to as a Mobitz Type I block, or the Wenckebach syndrome (see Fig. 7). In those instances where the PR interval remains constant with an intermittant loss of a QRS compex, then the block is termed a Mobitz Type II block (Ettinger, 1983). When three or more subsequent atrial impulses are blocked in a row, then the term 'advanced' second degree AV block is employed.

Third degree AV blocks rarely occur spontaneously during anaesthesia. They are diagnosed electrocardiographically when no electrical conduction occurs through the AV node. Atrioventricular dissociation exists in this situation and there is no relationship between the P waves and QRS complexes (see Fig. 8). In the cat, third degree AV block of congenital origin occurs and is characterized by a relatively normal QRS conformation and ventricular rate. This is because the rhythm is usually initiated at the AV junction or in the bundle of His (Fox *et al.*, 1983). If a third degree AV block is acquired, the QRS complex is usually abnormal in configuration and the ventricular rate is low.

First degree heart blocks do not result in significant haemodynamic alteration. Mobitz Type I blocks are benign, readily treated and do not often result in significant intraoperative cardiovascular disturbances. Mobitz Type II blocks, on the other hand, are usually associated with disease of the His–Purkinje system and can readily progress to a complete heart block with a slow ventricular rate. Anaesthesia should not be induced in animals with a third degree heart block unless an artificial pacemaker is available.

Heart blocks may occur as the result of: (1) congenital abnormalities; (2) toxins from infectious processes; (3) acquired heart disease; (4) cardiac trauma; (5) increased vagal tone; (6) hypoxia;

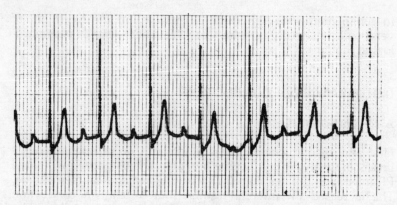

Fig. 6 First degree AV block is characterized by a prolonged PR interval.

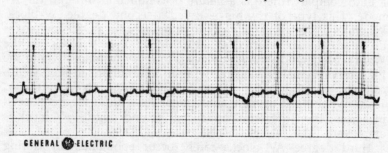

GENERAL ELECTRIC

Fig. 7 Second degree AV block (Mobitz Type I) is characterized by the loss of a QRS complex following a normal P wave.

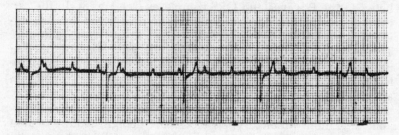

Fig. 8 Third degree AV block is characterized by complete dissociation of the P waves and QRS complexes.

(7) preanaesthetic agents, such as xylazine; (8) anaesthetic agents, such as halothane; (9) digitialis; and (10) electrolyte abnormalities.

First degree heart blocks and Mobitz Type I heart blocks are readily treated with anticholinergics, such as atropine, or adrenergic agents, such as isoprenaline (see Table 1). Mobitz Type II

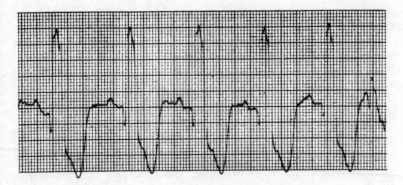

Fig. 9 Bundle branch block is characterized by a widened, often notched QRS complex. In this instance a left bundle branch block is characterized by aberrant conduction with positive QRS complexes.

blocks and third degree heart blocks do not usually respond to pharmacological therapy and a pacemaker is required to ensure adequate cardiac function during the perioperative period. Transoesophageal pacemakers are now commercially available and should be considered for use in clinical practice (Backofen *et al.*, 1984).

Bundle branch blocks

Bundle branch blocks which develop spontaneously during anaesthesia are rare. When these blocks do occur, they are a result of an impairment, or block, of the conduction system in one or more fascicles of the conduction system distal to the bundle of His. The result is an alteration of the normal sequence of impulses spread from the ventricular septum to either the right or left ventricles (Pratila, Pratilas and Dimich, 1979; Domino *et al.*, 1984).

Bundle branch blocks are recognized as bizarre QRS complexes that occur in association with a normal P wave and PR interval. The QRS complex is widened and may resemble an M or W in configuration or have a notch in the complex (see Fig. 9). Bundle branch blocks should be differentiated from the ventricular pre-excitation syndrome, where abnormal pathways connect the atrial muscle to ventricular muscle. The electrocardioscopic diagnosis of bundle branch blocks is discussed in detail by Ettinger and Suter (1970) and Tilley (1985).

In general, right and left bundle branch blocks are considered to have little effect on cardiovascular stability (Haft, Herman and Gorlin, 1971; Fox *et al.*, 1983; Tilley, 1985). However, on occasion, significant alterations in haemodynamic stability do occur especially if there is concurrent primary cardiac disease.

The causes of bundle branch blocks detected prior to anaesthesia are numerous and are listed elsewhere (Fox *et al.*, 1983; Tilley, 1985). Bundle branch blocks which occur spontaneously during anaesthesia are considered to be a rate-related aberrancy in man (Pratila *et al.*, 1979; Domino *et al.*, 1984). This rhythm disturbance is thought to be the result of small changes in cycle length that are too small to be diagnosed easily with a surface ECG. In order to diagnose a rate-dependent aberrancy, the atypical RR intervals must be recorded on a long strip and compared to the normal RR interval which was present earlier (Fisch, Zipps and McHenry, 1973).

If there are significant clinical effects as the result of a bundle branch block, treatment may be necessary. If the block is the result of an increase in heart rate over a critical value, vagal manoeuvre may be attempted with caution or neostigmine can be administered. (Domino *et al.*, 1984). Cardiac pacing is indicated in symptomatic left bundle branch blocks or in those which occur with a second degree AV block (Atlee, 1980).

Isorhythmic AV dissociation

This dysrhythmia may occur intraoperatively in patients with enhanced vagal tone when they are deeply anaesthetized with a potent inhalent agent (Atlee, 1980, 1984). Characteristically, the atrial rhythm is electrically related and set in some unknown fashion by the idioventricular rhythm. The ventricle maintains the dominant rhythm. The term synchrony implies that the atrial and ventricular rates are similar for long periods of time and that the P wave maintains a constant relationship to the QRS complex (Atlee, 1980). Accrochage refers to the phenomenon whereby the atrial and the ventricular rates are almost identical, but the P wave moves in and out of the QRS complex (Ettinger and Suter, 1970).

Isorhythmic AV dissociation may be distinguished from complete AV block by the normal appearance of the QRS complex and the constant relationship between the P waves and QRS complex (Atlee, 1980). On occasion it may also be associated with bradycardia resulting in severe hypotension. This is especially true if the anaesthetic is maintained with a potent inhalent agent such as halothane or enflurane.

If significant alterations in haemodynamic function occur, the plane of anaesthesia should be lightened. If hypotension is severe, consideration should be given to the administration of an adrenergic agonist such as ephedrine in conjunction with isotonic intravenous fluids (see Table 1). Recently it has been suggested that calcium chloride may be of value in the treatment of isorhythmic dissociation (Gottlieb *et al.*, 1986). Atropine should be avoided since it may result in the onset of more serious dysrhythmias.

CARDIAC ARREST

Cardiac arrest is often described as a five-minute emergency. Recent work in primates, however, has demonsrated that cardio-pulmonary resuscitation (CPR) is effective in restoring circulation for up to 12 min after arrest (Gilroy *et al.*, 1980). It is interesting to note that, while the cardiovascular system initially responded to therapy, only 53% of the animals survived 96 h or more (Gilroy *et al.*, 1980). In the majority of the survivors, impairment of the central nervous system was evident (Gilroy *et al.*, 1980). It is imperative that all cases are closely monitored during general anaesthesia so that the clinical signs of impending arrest can be recognized early and treated appropriately. Signs which could signal the onset of cardiac arrest include: (1) progressive or persistent tachy- or bradydysrhythmias; (2) conduction abnormal-ities; (3) uni- or multifocal ventricular extrasystoles; (4) persistent hypotension; (5) sudden ventilatory changes; and (6) cyanosis. The classical signs of cardiac arrest include: (1) absence of heart sounds; (2) lack of a peripheral pulse; (3) reduced bleeding at the surgical site; (4) apnoea; and (5) electrocardiographic evidence of asytole, ventricular fibrillation, electromechanical dissociation or an idioventricular rhythm.

The implementation of basic CPR is essential in cardiac arrest. However, a differential ECG diagnosis must be obtained rapidly so that the appropriate pharmacological therapy can be initiated. Asystole, the final common pathway of all forms of arrest, is characterized by the absence of electrical activity and myocardial contractions. In this case, the ECG presents as a straight line. The other electrocardiographic forms of arrest are illustrated in Figs. 10 to 12. Whatever the electrical diagnosis, effective cardiac output ceases and the clinical signs of cardiac arrest are evident.

While the only sensible approach to cardiac arrest is one of prevention, arrests do occur during anaesthesia, and it is possible to treat them successfully. For a detailed exposition of the phar-macological management of cardiac arrest, the reader is referred to the work of Crowe (1984) or any of the standard veterinary medical textbooks.

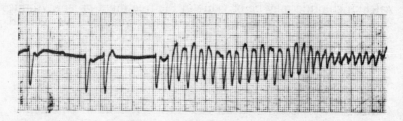

Fig. 10 Ventricular fibrillation may present in a fine, moderate or coarse pattern. In this illustration isolated ventricular escape beats progress to ventricular flutter and finally ventricular fibrillation.

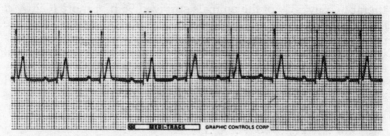

Fig. 11 Electromechanical dissociation may present as a relatively normal tracing with loss of cardiac output.

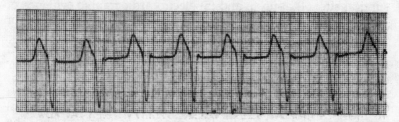

Fig. 12 Pulseless idioventricular rhythms are characterized by widened, bizarre QRS complexes.

REFERENCES

Alexander, J. W., Bolton, G. R. and Koslow, G. L. (1975). *Journal of the American Animal Hospital Association* **11**, 160.

Atlee, J. L. (1980). In *Anesthesia and the Patient with Heart Disease*, p. 137. Philadelphia: F. A. Davis Company.

Atlee, J. L. (1984). In *1984 Annual Refresher Course Lectures*, p. 202. Park Ridge, Ill.: American Society of Anesthesiologists.

Atlee, J. L. and Flaherty, M. P. (1983). *Anesthesiology* **59**, A84.

Atlee, J. L. and Malkinson, C. E. (1980). *Anesthesiology* **53**, S133.

Backofen, J. E., Schauble, J. F. and Rogers, M. C. (1984). *Anesthesiology* **61**, 777.

Bonagura, J. D. and Muir, M. W. (1985). In *Essentials of Canine and Feline Electrocardiography: Interpretation and Treatment*, 2nd edn, p. 281. Philadelphia: Lea and Febiger.

Corday, E. & Lang, T. W. (1974). In *The Heart Arteries and Veins*, p. 498. New York: McGraw-Hill.

Crowe, D. T. (1984). In *Veterinary Tauma and Critical Care*, p. 507. Philadelphia: Lea and Febiger.

Crowe, D. T. & Calvert, C.A. (1984). In *Veterinary Trauma and Critical Care*, p. 121. Philadelphia: Lea and Febiger.

Domino, K. B., La Mantina, K. L., Greer, R. T. and Klineberg, P. L. (1984). *Canadian Anaesthetists Society Journal* **31**, 302.

Ettinger, S. J. (1983). In *Textbook of Veterinary Internal Medicine*, p. 980, 2nd edn. Philadelphia: W. B. Saunders Company.

Ettinger, S. J. and Suter, P. F. (1970) In *Canine Cardiology*, p. 271. Philadelphia: W. B. Saunders Company.

Fisch, C., Zipps, D. P., and McHenry, P. L. (1973). *Circulation* **XLVIII**, 714.

Fox, P. R., Tilly, L. P. and Liu, S. K. (1983). In *Feline Medicine*, p. 249, 1st edn. Santa Barbara: American Veterinary Publications.

Gilroy, B. A., Rockoff, M. A., Dunlop, B. J. and Shapiro, H. M. (1980). *Journal of the American Veterinary Medical Association* **177**, 867.

Gottlieb, A., Satarino, P., Stehna, D. and Millar, R. A. (1986). *Anesthesiology* **64**, 407.

Haft, J. I., Herman, M. V. and Gorlin, R. (1971). *Circulation* **XLIII**, 279.

Hubbell, J. A. E., Muir, W. W., Bednarski, R. M. and Bednarski, L. S. (1984). *Journal of the American Veterinary Medical Association* **185**, 643.

Joas, T. A. and Stevens, W. C. (1971). *Anesthesiology* **35**, 48.

Johnson, J. T. (1985). *Journal of the American Animal Hospital Association* **21**, 429.

Klide, A. M., Calderwood, H. W. and Soma, L. R. (1975). *American Journal of Veterinary Research* **36**, 931.

Maze, M. and Smith, C. M. (1983). *Anesthesiology* **59**, 322.

Maze, M. and Smith, C. M. (1985). *Journal of the American Veterinary Medical Association* **186**, 648.

Metz, S. and Maze, M. (1985). *Anesthesiology* **62**, 470.

Muir, W. W. (1977a). *Journal of the American Veterinary Medical Association* **170**, 1419.

Muir, W. W. (1977b). *American Journal of Veterinary Research* **38**, 1377.

Muir, W. W. (1978). *Journal of the American Veterinary Medical Association* **172**, 917.

Muir, W. W., Werner, L. L. and Hamlin, R. L. (1975). *American Journal of Veterinary Research* **36**, 1299.

Munson, E. S. and Tucker, W. K. (1975). *Canadian Anaesthetists Society Journal* **22**, 495.

Musselman, E. (1976). *Journal of the American Veterinary Medical Association* **168**, 145.

Pratila, M. G., Pratilas, V. and Dimich, I. (1979). *Anesthesiology* **51**, 461.

Spiss, C. K., Maze, M. and Smith, C. M. (1983). *Anesthesiology* **59**, A83.

Stahl, W. R. (1967). *Journal of Applied Physiology* **22**, 453.

Stoelting, R. K. and Miller, R. D. (1984). In *Basics of Anesthesia*, p. 43. New York: Churchill Livingstone.

Sumikawa, K., Ishizaka, N. and Suzaki, M. (1983). *Anesthesiology* **58**, 322.

Tilley, L. P. (1985). In *Essentials of Canine and Feline Electrocardiography: Interpretation and Treatment*, 2nd edn, p. 55. Philadelphia: Lea and Febiger.

Wit, A. L. and Rosen, M. R. (1983). *American Heart Journal* **106**, 798.

7

The clinical pharmacology of agents used to manage cardiovascular instability during anaesthesia

Recommended techniques for safe anaesthesia of small animal patients emphasize the importance of closely monitoring cardiovascular function (Soma, 1974; Dodman, Seeler and Court, 1984). Minimum acceptable standards for safe anaesthetic practice mandate that heart rate and peripheral pulse should be monitored periodically during anaesthesia. More sophisticated cardiovascular monitoring includes electrocardioscopic evaluation of heart rate and rhythm in addition to measurement of systemic arterial pressure. If detected early, many causes of haemodynamic instability can be corrected by relatively subtle alterations in anaesthetic technique and the use of specific pharmacological agents may not be required (Dodman, Seeler and Court, 1984). Failure of conservative measures to control potentially insidious dysrhythmias is an indication for the use of pharmacological therapy. In these instances it is important to be familiar with agents which can be used intraoperatively, to have agents available and to have rapid access to or knowledge of effective dose rates and possible adverse sequelae. This chapter will list available agents and review their clinical pharmacology. It will include discussion of conventional antidysrhythmic drugs, other agents with antidysrhythmic properties, agents affecting the autonomic system, and inotropic agents.

ANTIDYSRHYTHMIC AGENTS

Antidysrhythmic agents are traditionally grouped into four classes according to their electrophysiological properties (Vaughan Williams, 1984). Class 1 antidysrhythmics consist of the sodium

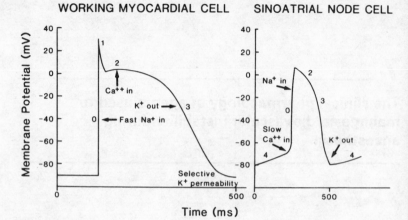

Fig. 1 In the working myocardial cell, the resting membrane potential is maintained at a constant level by a balanced influx and efflux of K^+. At the time of excitation of the membrane, there is a rapid Na^+ influx through fast Na^+ channels and a sharp rate of rise of phase 0 of the action potential. During phase 2, the membrane potential is partly restored by an influx of Ca^{2+} through the slowly conducting Ca^{2+} channels. It is this influx of Ca^{2+} that stimulates greater release of Ca^{2+} from myocardial stores and allows myocellular contraction. In contrast, the resting membrane potential of the sinoatrial nodal cells drifts upwards. The rate of phase 0 is slower owing to (1) the less negative membrane potential at the time of excitation and (2) the participation of Ca^{2+} in the early part of phase 0. Class 1 agents reduce the maximum rate and amplitude of depolarization of phase 0 of the action potential of the working myocardial cell. Class 2 agents have no specific effects on the action potential. Class 3 agents prolong the action potential duration (APD) and effective refractory period (ERP). Class 4 agents inhibit the influx of Ca^{2+} during phases 0 and 2, especially in pacemaker cells.

channel blockers. Blockade of sodium channels reduces the maximum rate and amplitude of depolarization in phase 0 of the cardiac action potential and, as a consequence, the conduction velocity is slowed (Fig. 1). The automaticity of the His–Purkinje system is also decreased. The sinoatrial (SA) and atrioventricular (AV) nodes are unaffected by therapeutic plasma concentrations of class 1 antidysrhythmics because these nodes have an action potential dependent on a calcium current for depolarization rather than a sodium influx.

Class 1a antidysrhythmics delay membrane repolarization by prolonging the action potential duration (APD) and the effective refractory period (ERP) in both normal and injured myocardial tissue. Unidirectional conduction blocks are usually converted to

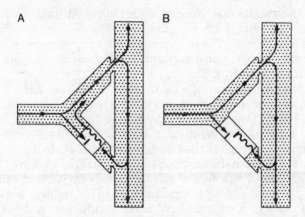

Fig. 2 (A) Diagrammatic representation of the path taken by myocardial electrical impulses during re-entrant dysrhythmias in damaged myocardial cells. Stippled areas indicate zones of normal myocardial cell function. The open area represents a damaged portion of myocardial fibre. (B) The effect of class 1a and 1b antidysrhythmics on electrical impulse conduction in damaged myocardial cells.

bidirectional blocks by class 1a drugs, thus interrupting re-entry mechanisms (Fig. 2). Class 1b agents eliminate re-entry by either depressing conduction and converting unidirectional blocks into bidirectional blocks or eliminating the block (Donegan, 1986). The former situation usually applies to damaged myocardial cells and the latter to normal myocardial tissue (Fig. 2). In contrast to 1a drugs, 1b drugs have almost no effect on the APD and ERP of normal myocardial cells (Adams, 1986). An increase in the dispersion of refractoriness is common following myocardial ischaemia. Lignocaine reduces the dispersion, stabilizes the myocardium and elevates the electrophysiological threshold for ventricular fibrillation (Atlee, 1985; Donegan, 1986).

The sodium blocking activity of class 1 antidysrhythmics is affected by alterations in plasma potassium concentration and plasma pH. Extracellular potassium levels less than 4.5 mEq l^{-1} substantially reduce the effect of therapeutic concentrations of lignocaine while potassium levels exceeding 6.0 mEq l^{-1} may result in manifestations of lignocaine toxicity at therapeutic concentrations (Atlee, 1985). Therefore, serum potassium levels must be corrected for the safe and efficacious use of lignocaine.

Class 2 antidysrhythmics comprise the beta-adrenoceptor antagonists and, as such, produce their most profound effects in the presence of elevated sympathetic tone. β-Adrenoceptor blockade reduces the rate of automaticity in the SA node and Purkinje fibres. The conduction velocity through the AV node is reduced and the APD and ERP are increased. The ERP of the Purkinje fibres is lengthened. The membrane stabilizing properties of these agents are clinically insignificant at therapeutic plasma levels (Bonagura and Muir, 1985).

The pharmacological agents in class 3 do not directly affect automaticity or conduction velocity. Their major action is to prolong the APD and ERP by directly delaying membrane repolarization, especially in ventricular and Purkinje fibres. Some antiadrenergic properties of class 3 agents are also evident.

Class 4 antidysrhythmics, the calcium channel or slow channel inhibitors, limit the influx of calcium across excitable membranes during phases 0 and 2 of depolarization. This reduces the availability of calcium for SA and AV nodal conduction and SA nodal automaticity (Merin, 1981; Adams, 1982). At therapeutic levels, verapamil has no effect on the conduction velocity or resting membrane potential in normal atrial, ventricular or Purkinje fibres since the electrical activity of these fibres relies on sodium channel function rather than calcium channel function. Myocardial contractility and peripheral myogenic activity in vascular smooth muscle are decreased. Verapamil, diltiazem and nifedipine are probably the best known members of class 4. Verapamil and diltiazem are the most effective antidysrhythmics of this group. Nifedipine has negligible cardiac electrophysiological effects at clinically useful doses (Atlee, 1985).

Class (1a) antidysrhythmics

Procainamide hydrochloride (Pronestyl). Procainamide is used in the management of ventricular dysrhythmias. A 90% success rate has been reported in the treatment of premature ventricular depolarizations and paroxysmal ventricular tachycardias in man (Bigger, 1980). Acute atrial fibrillation and flutter may also respond to procainamide therapy although higher doses are required (Bonagura and Muir, 1985). Although the indications for procainamide therapy are similar to those for quinidine therapy, procainamide is preferred for intravenous use because it has fewer adverse cardiovascular effects (Atlee, 1985).

Slow intravenous administration of procainamide at doses less than 10 mg kg^{-1} produces little change in cardiac output, myocardial contractility or left ventricular end diastolic pressures (Bonagura and Muir, 1985). The heart rate may increase and there is a slight decrease in blood pressure and total peripheral resistance. These effects are associated with the anticholinergic and ganglion blocking activities of procainamide (Bonagura and Muir, 1985).

Electrocardiographic changes are insignificant over the clinical dose range.

The therapeutic plasma range of procainamide in dogs is 4–10 μg ml^{-1} (Davis, 1984). Twenty per cent of an intravenously administered dose is bound to plasma protein. The elimination half-life is approximately 2.5 hours in the dog with biliary excretion being the major route of elimination (Bonagura and Muir, 1985). N-Acetylprocainamide is the major cardioactive metabolite in man, but only minute quantities have been identified in dogs and cats (Bonagura and Muir, 1985).

Toxic effects encountered with procainamide administration include myocardial depression, hypotension, prolonged PR, QRS and QT intervals, AV blocks and ventricular tachydysrhythmias. All of these symptoms are associated with rapid intravenous administratioin of the drug or excessive doses. When treating atrial fibrillation, slowing of the atrial rate by procainamide therapy may adversely raise the ventricular rate by improving AV nodal conduction. Procainamide can severely depress myocardial function in dogs with sick sinus syndrome, and its use is contraindicated if idioventricular rhythm exists (Bonagura and Muir, 1985).

Quinidine (Kinidin, Quinicardine). Quinidine resembles procainamide in its spectrum of antidysrhythmic activities. It is sometimes used in an attempt to control intraoperative atrial fibrillation, but dangerously high doses may be rquired and DC cardioversion is the preferred treatment. Quinidine therapy for atrial fibrillation may produce either sinus rhythm or atrial flutter. Conversion to a sinus rhythm occurs in about 10–20% of human patients and is most likely to occur if the fibrillation is of recent onset and there is no atrial enlargement (Atlee, 1985). Slow intravenous administration of quinidine gluconate in the clinical dose range of 1.0–5.0 mg kg^{-1} does not usually alter myocardial function although α-adrenoceptor blockade and resultant hypotension are common sequelae.

The therapeutic plasma concentration of quinidine ranges from 2.5 to 5.0 μg ml^{-1} (Davis, 1984). Quinidine is 80% protein bound in dogs and 85% protein bound in cats (Davis, 1984; Bonagura and Muir, 1985). Eighty per cent of quinidine undergoes hepatic metabolism prior to renal excretion with the elimination half-life being 5.6 hours in the dog and 1.9 hours in the cat (Davis, 1984). The extent of antidysrhythmic activity possessed by the metabolites has not been determined in the canine and feline species (Bonagura and Muir, 1985). Quinidine is a potent inhibitor of hepatic microsomal enzymes and may increase the duration of action of other drugs which are metabolized by the liver.

The blood pressure and electrocardiogram should be monitored continuously during intravenous quinidine therapy. Signs of over-dosage include reduced AV nodal conduction, heart block, atrial standstill and ventricular fibrillation. The QRS complex may widen or SA and AV nodel conduction disturbances may appear. Quinidine elevates the plasma levels of digoxin and digitoxin and potentiates the action of non-depolarizing muscle relaxants (Atlee, 1985). Rarely, anaphylaxis results from quinidine administration (Atlee, 1985).

Class 1b antidysrhythmics

Lignocaine hydrochloride (Xlyocaine). Lignocaine is commonly used to treat acute intraoperative ventricular dysrhythmias because it is effective, well tolerated and has a rapid onset of action when administered intravenously (Anderson, 1984). At therapeutic levels, lignocaine produces minimal change in ventricular contractility, cardiac output, arterial pressure or heart rate. Coronary blood flow increases. The electrocardiogram is rarely affected by therapeutic plasma levels of lignocaine although the QT interval may be shortened. At plasma levels which are toxic, the QRS complex may be widened (Anderson, 1984; Davis, 1984; Bonagura and Muir, 1985).

The therapeutic plasma range in dogs is between 2 and 6 μg ml^{-1} (Davis, 1984). Approximately 70% of an administered dose of lignocaine is bound to plasma protein. The elimination half-life is approximately 1.0–1.5 hours in the dog, although liver and cardiac failure can reduce its clearance from plasma (Bonagura and Muir, 1985). Liver metabolism produces active and inactive metabolites and when monitoring plasma lignocaine levels, the active metabolites should be considered. About 5% of an administered dose is excreted unchanged in the urine.

The use of lignocaine is contraindicated in patients with sick sinus syndrome, second or third degree heart block, idioventricular rhythms, and in patients with sinus bradycardia accompanied by ventricular escape beats. Hypotension and negative inotropic and chronotropic cardiac effects may occur when plasma levels of the parent drug and its active metabolites exceed 8 μg ml^{-1} (Adams, 1982; Wilcke, 1985). Many of the common clinical signs of lignocaine toxicity such as nausea, disorientation, depression, neuromuscular excitability and convulsions often occur with intravenous boluses exceeding 4 mg kg^{-1} but they may be masked by anaesthesia. Other signs such as respiratory depression or arrest will be evident (Adams, 1982). Cats are very susceptible to lignocaine-induced seizures, possibly due to a local anaesthetic-induced reduction in release of gamma-aminobutyric acid, a central inhibitory neurotransmitter (Ikeda, Dohi and Tsujimoto, 1983). An alternative explanation for seizures is selective depression or inhibitory cortical neurons (Tanaka & Tamasaki, 1966).

Aprinidine. Aprinidine has been used experimentally in dogs. It has been found to be highly effective in the treatment of refractory ventricular dysrhythmias at intravenous doses of 0.5–2.0 mg kg^{-1}. It has a narrow therapeutic index and potential adverse effects include leucopenia, hepatopathy, convulsions, transient depression of myocardial contractility and polymorphous ventricular tachycardia. Its use can presently only be recommended as a last resort (Atlee 1985; Bonagura and Muir, 1985).

Class 2 antidysrhythmics

Propranolol hydrochloride (Inderal). The major indication for the use of propranolol is in the management of supraventricular dysrhythmias such as atrial premature depolarizations and paroxysmal supraventricular tachycardias or junctional tachycardias. Atrial fibrillation and atrial flutter occasionally respond favourably to the administration of propranolol, especially if a high degree of sympathetic tone is present. Increased sympathetic tone is common with hyperthyroidism or when stressful procedures are performed under light anaesthesia (Adams, 1982; Bonagura and Muir, 1985). Propranolol has been combined with digitalis to control the ventricular rate in atrial fibrillation when digitalis alone is ineffective (Muir and Sams, 1984). Together, these two agents considerably slow conduction through the AV node thus reducing the ventricular rate and improving cardiac output. A combination of propranolol and quinidine has been used to convert atrial fibrillation to sinus rhythm, but the efficacy and safety of this regimen is still unproven (Bonagura and Muir, 1985).

Propranolol has limited use in the treatment of ventricular dysrhythmias except in the cat, where it will often control ventricular tachycardia. Ventricular dysrhythmias triggered by high sympathetic tone usually respond to low doses of the drug.

In addition to its antidysrhythmic properties, propranolol has several other cardiovascular effects. Cardiac contractility, cardiac output, myocardial oxygen consumption and arterial blood pressure fall. The total peripheral resistance may reflexly increase (Atlee, 1985; Bonagura and Muir, 1985). The heart rate slows and this increases the time available for myocardial perfusion during diastole. The risk of myocardial ischaemia is therefore reduced (Muir and Sams, 1984).

The therapeutic plasma level of propranolol in the dog is 40–120 ng ml^{-1} (Davis, 1984). Propranolol is extensively bound to plasma protein, especially α_1 acid glycoprotein and albumin. Elevation of the plasma level of α_1 acid glycoprotein during chronic inflammation or heart failure decreases the half-life of propranolol (Bonagura and Muir, 1985). The elimination half-life of propranolol in the normal dog is in the range of 30 minutes to 1 hour in the dog and 30 minutes in the cat (Bonagura and Muir, 1985). Propranolol undergoes rapid hepatic metabolism and the plasma clearance of this drug closely approaches hepatic blood flow. It may reduce its own clearance by reducing cardiac output and subsequently reducing hepatic blood flow (Muir and Sams, 1984). Metabolites of propranolol have not been shown to have any appreciable clinical effect after administration to normal dogs but may become significant when there is renal impairment (Muir and Sams, 1984). The pharmacological response to propranolol therapy is proportional to the existing sympathetic tone. Accordingly, the initial dose should be given slowly and to effect.

The incidence of adverse reactions to propranolol administration appears to be unrelated to dose. It is high in geriatric animals with heart failure or azotaemia (Muir and Sams, 1984). Adverse reactions include hypotension, bradycardia, heart block, aggravation of congestive heart failure, bronchospasm and occasional hypoglycaemia. Clinical signs of toxicity are mostly the result of β-adrenoceptor blockade although a rapid bolus injection can produce non-specific cardiovascular depression (Adams, 1982). In patients with left ventricular failure, a high level of sympathetic activity maintains cardiac output. In this instance β-adrenoceptor blockade may lead to acute cardiovascular collapse. Occasionally, propranolol precipitates left ventricular failure in the absence of known previous cardiac disease. The sudden withdrawal from chronic propranolol medication is sometimes recommended as a preoperative measure but can induce cardiac disorders such as tachycardia, dysrhythmias and hypertension (Muir and Sams, 1984). Chronic propranolol administration should therefore be terminated by reducing the dosage in a stepwise fashion over several days.

Class 3 antidysrhythmics

Bretylium tosylate (Bretylate). In man, bretylium is used to treat refractory ventricular tachydysrhythmias and recurrent ventricular fibrillation. However, it has had only very limited success in veterinary medicine and furthermore can precipitate ventricular tachycardia and fibrillation (Bonagura and Muir, 1985). Currently, its use cannot be recommended in veterinary patients.

Following intravenous administration, bretylium is taken up by the sympathetic ganglia and nerve terminals where it causes an initial release of catecholamines. This is associated with a transient rise in cardiac output, contractility and blood pressure. Later, catecholamine release is prevented and these parameters are depressed (Bonagura and Muir, 1985). The sympathetic activities of bretylium may be at least partly responsible for its antidysrhythmic properties but there is also evidence that bretylium reduces the dispersion of the APD and ERP in normal and infarcted canine Purkinje fibres (Atlee, 1985). The pharmacokinetics of bretylium in the dog and the cat have yet to be reported.

Because bretylium causes a transient release of catecholamines, is use with halogenated anaesthetics may be contraindicated (Novotny and Adams, 1986).

Amiodarone hydrochloride. Amiodarone, a benzofurane which is structurally related to thyroxine, has been used as a vasodilator for the treatment of coronary arterial spasm in man for several years. It has recently been used in the clinical management of recurrent ventricular tachycardias in man. Amiodarone has both α- and β-adrenoceptor blocking properties. Sinus nodal automaticity and conduction time are depressed and there is increased refractoriness within the atria, AV node and ventricles. Conduction is slowed through the AV node and His-Purkinje system, but not in atrial and ventricular muscle fibres (Atlee, 1985). Early reports of its intraoperative use in man are not encouraging, as both hypotension and atropine-resistant bradycardia have been reported to occur after its use during general anaesthesia (Feinberg, La Mantia and Levy, 1986).

Class 4 antidysrhythmics

Verapamil (Cordilox). In man, verapamil is used in the management of supraventricular tachydysrhythmias. It is also used to slow the ventricular rate during atrial flutter or fibrillation. In veterinary medicine verapamil has still to be adequately assessed and should be used cautiously. Intravenous administration of verapamil in dogs has been associated with negative inotropic effects and peripheral and coronary vasodilatation (Drop, 1985). Cardiovascular depression can be dangerously profound if this drug is used in combination with higher therapeutic doses of halothane, isoflurane or enflurane (Chelly *et al.*, 1986a, b). After intravenous administration, AV block occurs within minutes and prolonged conduction through this node persists for up to 6 hours. The degree of AV nodal block reflects plasma levels of verapamil. Electrocardiographically, the PR interval is prolonged. In dogs, intravenous doses range from 50 to 150 μg kg^{-1} and are administered over 5 minutes followed by an infusion of 2–10 μg kg^{-1} min^{-1}

(Novotny and Adams, 1986). The elimination half-time of verapa-mil in the dog is approximately 1-6 hours with activity being terminated by extensive hepatic metabolism.

Verapamil overdose causes severe AV nodal depression with consequent second and third degree heart blocks, hypotension, and even asystole (Wilcke, 1985). Pre-existing heart blocks, bradycardia and sick sinus syndrome are contraindications to the use of verapa-mil. Marked hypotension and even cardiogenic shock have been reported in dogs with cardiomyopathy and atrial fibrillation in which verapamil therapy was instituted (Bonagura and Muir, 1985).

Digitalis glycosides—digoxin (Diganox, Lanoxin), digitoxin

The role of digitalis glycosides as inotropic agents in the intraopera-tive setting is limited but they may be required to reduce the ventricular rate during atrial fibrillation or flutter (Rinke, 1986). These drugs improve contractility in both the normal and failing heart. Current theories suggest that digoxin inhibits the Na^+-K^+ ATP-ase pump allowing sodium ions to accumulate within the cardiac cell. This encourages exchange of sodium for calcium ions across the myocardial membrane (Adams, 1982). The increased intracellular concentration of calcium rises and contractility is improved. In the failing heart, digitalis glycosides improve contrac-tility and cardiac outflow without necessarily increasing myocardial oxygen consumption (Adams, 1982). In-vivo antidysrhythmic activ-ities ascribed to this group of drugs are mostly due to indirect effects. As cardiac output and function improve, reflex sympathetic activity is reduced. Vagal tone is elevated by digitalis preparations tending to reduce the sinus rate, increase the refractory period and reduce conduction velocity at the AV node (Adams, 1982).

Several factors influence the response to digitalis glycosides. Atropine, for example, will oppose the vagal effects. Hypoxaemia, fever, sepsis and trauma decrease the extent to which the heart rate is reduced (Davis, 1984). The presence of hypercalcaemia, elevated intracellular potassium levels, hypokalaemia, hypomag-nesaemia, hypoxaemia, renal failure, chronic pulmonary disease or acute myocardial infarction increases the risk of toxicity with digitalis glycosides.

The pharmacology and pharmacokinetics of the digitalis drugs are well documented elsewhere (Davis, 1984). The effective plasma level range of digoxin is between 0.5 and 2.0 mg ml^{-1} (Adams, 1982). The elimination half-life is 15-23 hours in dogs and up to 33 hours in cats (Bonagura and Muir, 1985). Of particular note is the low therapeutic index of the digitalis preparations. The minimum effective plasma concentration is approximately 70% of the toxic plasma concentration in the healthy animal (Davis, 1984). It may take up to 60 minutes for maximal positive inotropic responses to be observed following intravenous administration, making these agents very difficult and dangerous to titrate effectively if given intravenously (Hamlin, Dutta and Smith, 1971).

Signs of digoxin toxicity relate to the cardiovascular, central nervous and gastrointestinal systems. Prominent cardiovascular signs include heart block, premature ventricular contractions, ventricular tachycardia and in extreme situations ventricular fibrillation (Davis, 1984; Bonagura and Muir, 1985). Digitalization should not be attempted in patients with any of these conditions.

DRUGS ACTING ON ADRENERGIC RECEPTORS

β_1-Adrenoceptors predominate in the heart. In the SA node, β-adrenoceptor agonists produce positive chronotrophy, resulting from an accelerated opening of calcium channels. Within the AV node, conduction velocity is increased (positive dromotropy) and conduction is improved in the Purkinje fibre network (Katz, 1977). In the ventricular myocardium, activation of β-adrenoceptors enhances the activity of adenylate cyclase, increasing production of cyclic adenosine monophosphate. This increases the calcium influx and calcium availability in the myoplasm (Prys-Roberts, 1980). Cardiac contractility is then improved. Positive chronotropic, dromotropic and inotropic effects of cardiac adrenoceptor stimulation are associated with a considerable increase in myocardial oxygen consumption (Chernow, Rainery and Lake, 1982).

α-Adrenoceptors have been identified in atrial tissue, but the clinical significance of these findings has not yet been fully elucidated (Lawson and Wallfische, 1986). Peripherally, α-adrenoceptor stimulation causes vasoconstriction. β-Adrenoceptor mediated vasodilatation occurs in arterioles supplying coronary, pulmonary and skeletal muscle.

Agonists

Adrenaline (Simplene). During anaesthesia, adrenaline is used to treat asystole, cardiogenic shock and drug hypersensitivity reactions. It should only be used in critical patients and only then if safer adrenergic agents have failed. The exception to this rule is asystolic cardiac arrest when adrenaline is the agent of choice. Fine fibrillation which is refractory to cardioversion may be converted to coarse fibrillation with adrenaline, thus improving the chances for cardioversion (Chernow *et al.*, 1982).

Adrenaline is a potent vasopressor and myocardial stimulant. It increases blood pressure by cardiac β-adrenoceptor agonism and, to a lesser extent, by stimulating peripheral α-adrenoceptors.

The plasma half-life of adrenaline in man ranges from 5 to 7 minutes due to rapid deactivation by the catechol-*o*-methytransferase system and monoamine oxidase system (Prys-Roberts, 1980). Inactive metabolites are excreted in the urine.

When administered rapidly intravenously, adrenaline has the potential to cause sudden death from ventricular dysrhythmias or cerebral haemorrhage. It should be used cautiously in patients with hyperthyroidism or cardiac dysrhythmias or when halogenated anaesthetic agents are being used. Adrenaline has a greater propensity to cause dysrhythmias than dopamine or dobutamine, and, in combination with halothane, will cause dysrhythmias at dosages within the limits suggested for treatment of cardiac failure (Bednarski and Muir, 1983).

Solutions of adrenaline, isoproterenol and dopamine are oxidized upon exposure to light, air or heat. Accordingly, adrenaline is supplied in brown bottles and should be stored in cool locations out of direct light. Adrenaline, like solutions of dopamine, dobutamine and isoproterenol, is inactivated by alkaline solutions.

Isoprenaline (Aleudrin). Isoprenaline is used to induce cardiac acceleration and to manage heart blocks. Being a potent and β_2-adrenoceptor against it has positive chronotropic, dromotropic and inotropic effects, reduces arteriolar resistance, increases venous capacitance and usually causes significant hypotension (Lawson and Wallfische, 1986). It is rapidly metabolized by the catecholamine transferase system and has a short duration of action. Isoprenaline should be used cautiously since its intense chronotropic and inotropic effects substantially increase myocardial oxygen consumption and dysrhythmias occur readily. Excessive doses can cause cardiac necrosis secondary to ischaemia as oxygen demand exceeds the coronary artery supply. Its use is contraindicated in patients with hyperthyroidism or digitalis toxicity.

Dopamine hydrochloride (Intropin). Indications for the intraoperative administration of dopamine include bradycardia which is refractory to atropine and shock syndromes involving circulatory maldistribution such as septic and haemorrhagic shock (Chernow *et al.*, 1982; Crowe and Calvert, 1984; Lawson and Wallfische, 1986).

Dopamine stimulates adrenergic and dopaminergic receptors. At doses ranging from 0.5 to 2.0 μg kg^{-1} min^{-1} dopaminergic receptors in the renal, mesenteric, coronary and intracerebral blood vessels are selectively stimulated resulting in a fall in arterial resistance and blood pressure. At this low dose rate, venoconstriction occurs (Lawson and Wallfische, 1986). Myocardial chronotropy and inotropy are only slightly affected but cardiac output increases due to the reduced afterload and increased preload (Lawson and Wallfische, 1986). Diuresis and natriuresis resulting from inhibition of aldosterone synthesis and release occur (Chernow and Zolaga, 1987). At infusion rates between 2 and 10 μg kg^{-1} min^{-1}, the beta-one adrenoceptors are the primary target and myocardial contractility and cardiac output are improved with slight change in heart rate and blood pressure (Chernow *et al.*, 1982; Ogilvie, 1982). When 10–20 μg kg^{-1} min^{-1} are infused, both α_1- and β_1-adrenoceptors are activated with α_1-adrenoceptor activity predominating. Systemic blood pressure, pulmonary blood pressure, total peripheral resistance and heart rate all increase dramatically. Renal and mesenteric arteries also constrict. The overall cardiovascular response to dopamine is modified by a simultaneous noradrenaline response, since dopamine is capable of releasing endogenous noradrenaline (Merin, 1986). The release of noradrenaline increases the risk of ventricular dysrhythmias during dopamine therapy, especially in the presence of halogenated anaesthetics (Adams, 1982).

It is advisable to give the patient a loading dose of fluids before administering dopamine to avoid a hypotensive crisis. Because dopamine increases preload before increasing myocardial inotropy, its use may not be appropriate in heart failure when the ventricular filling pressure is already elevated. Under these circumstances, a further increase in ventricular wall tension may precipitate cardiac collapse. The use of dopamine is dangerous if tachydysrhythmias are present, although dopamine is less dysrhythmogenic in 'beta-range' doses than adrenaline (Chernow *et al.*, 1982).

Dobutamine hydrochloride (Dobutrex). Due to its inotropic properties, dobutamine is used for the management of congestive heart failure. It is not a conventional antidysrhythmic agent but does accelerate conduction through the AV node and therefore may be useful in the treatment of refractory second or third degree AV blocks.

Dobutamine, a synthetic catecholamine, was designed to selectively increase cardiac contractility without proportionally increasing heart rate or afterload (Adams, 1982). It has a negligible effect on venous tone (Chernow *et al.*, 1982; Lawson and Wallfische, 1986). Unlike dopamine, dobutamine is not a dopaminergic receptor agonist and so does not vasodilate in the renal, mesenteric, cerebral and coronary blood vessels. Also unlike dopamine, dobutamine does not stimulate or sensitize the myocardium by indirect noradrenaline release and is less likely than dopamine or adrenaline to cause dysrhythmias (Chernow *et al.*, 1982). The positive inotropic effects of dobutamine predominate when the infusion rate is between 2 and 10 μg kg^{-1} min^{-1} (Chernow *et al.*, 1982). At infusion rates greater than 10 μg kg^{-1} min^{-1}, tachydysrhythmias often occur (Chernow *et al.*, 1982). It should be used cautiously in patients with atrial fibrillation or flutter because it increases AV conduction and may cause an unacceptable increase in ventricular rate.

Antagonists

Conventional pharmacology of the adrenergic antagonists is found in most veterinary pharmacology texts and will not be included here. This section will briefly describe the role of these agents as investigational cardiac therapeutic drugs.

In recent years, it has become increasingly evident that sensitization of the heart to catecholamines by halothane is mediated not only by β-adrenoceptors but also by post-synaptic α-adrenoceptors (Maze and Smith, 1983). This may account for some of the antidysrhythmic activity demonstrated by specific α_1-adrenoceptor antagonists such as droperidol, acepromazine, prazosin and phentolamine (Muir, Werner and Hamlin, 1975; Maze and Smith, 1983). A number of cardiac dysrhythmias are sensitive to alterations in arterial blood pressure and indirect antidysrhythmic effects of α-adrenoceptor blocking agents are related to a reduction in cardiac afterload (Muir *et al.*, 1975; Bigger, 1980).

Although routine intraoperative use of α-adrenoceptor antagonists cannot yet be recommended, these new findings have implications for treatment of patients likely to suffer halothane–adrenaline interactions.

DRUGS ACTING ON CHOLINERGIC RECEPTORS

Parasympatholytics—atropine sulphate and glycopyrronium (Robinal)

Atropine and glycopyrronium (glycopyrrolate) are employed intraoperatively to treat sinus bradycardia. Some first and second degree AV blocks will also respond. The response to atropine depends on the extent of prevailing parasympathetic tone, the dose rate and rate of uptake into the systemic circulation. Intravenous doses of atropine exceeding 0.015 mg kg^{-1} increase the cardiac output by increasing heart rate (Adams, 1982). Arterial blood pressure remains unchanged or increases slightly in normal animals.

Occasionally, atropine administration will result in one of several unexpected effects. In low doses (0.015 mg kg^{-1} or less) or if uptake of the drug into the systemic circulation is prolonged, atropine may induce bradycardia. The mechanism is unclear but a weak peripheral muscarinic receptor effect of atropine has been implicated (Stoelting, 1987). Atropine exerts a differential effect on the SA and AV nodes, and second degree AV block and premature ventricular depolarizations can occur if this drug is given in low doses (Muir, 1978). Atropine may also indirectly exert sympathomimetic activity (Stoelting, 1987). The cardiac parasympathetic outflow normally suppresses production of noradrenaline during stimulation of cardiac sympathetic nerves (Muir, 1978). Atropine administration abolishes this protective mechanism and predisposes to dysrhythmias. Higher doses of atropine directly depress the myocardium (Adams, 1982).

Glycopyrronium at comparable dosages causes similar trends on heart rate to those of atropine although glycopyrronium has a longer activity onset time and a longer duration of action (Atlee, 1985). At therapeutic doses, tachycardia and intraoperative dysrhythmias are observed less frequently than with atropine (Mirakhur, 1979). Overall, glycopyrronium preserves cardiovascular stability better than atropine.

Parasympathomimetics—edrophonium chloride (Tensilon)

Edrophonium, an anticholinesterase, has been used as a treatment for paroxysmal supraventricular tachycardia and has been used to slow the ventricular rate in atrial flutter or fibrillation in man (Atlee, 1985). This drug has a rapid onset of action, a short duration and few adverse cardiovascular effects except for bradycardia. Information on the pharmacokinetics of edrophonium has been sparse due to difficulties in analytical techniques. Work in humans indicates that the half-life in normal patients is 100 minutes and that about 75% of elimination is by renal excretion (Miller and Savarese, 1986). Parasympathomimetics should be given cautiously to patients with cardiac failure, especially if heart blocks are present since they may induce sinus arrest, third degree AV block and rarely, asystole. These effects can be reversed with atropine.

Table 1. Dosages and infusion constants of emergency drugs

Procainamide hydrochloride (10%; 100 mg ml^{-1})
Bolus: dogs, 4–6 mg kg^{-1} i.v. slowly
Constant infusion
Rate: 10–40 μg kg^{-1} min^{-1}
Add: 2 ml (200 mg) to 500 ml 5% dextrose to give 400 μg/ml
Infuse 0.025–0.1 ml kg^{-1} min^{-1}

Quinidine gluconate (8%; 80 mg ml^{-1})
Bolus: 1.0–2.0 mg kg^{-1} slowly

Lignocaine hydrochloride (2%; 20 mg ml^{-1})
Bolus: dog, 1–4 mg kg^{-1} i.v.
      cat, 0.25–0.75 mg kg^{-1} i.v.

Constant infusion
Rate: 25–80 μg kg^{-1} min^{-1}
Add: 25 ml (500 mg) to 500 ml 5% dextrose to give 1000 μg ml^{-1}
Infuse 0.025–0.08 ml kg^{-1} min^{-1}

Propranolol hydrochloride (0.1%; 1 mg ml^{-1})
Bolus: 0.04–0.06 mg kg^{-1} slowly i.v.
Administer 1 mg min^{-1}

Adrenaline (1:1000; 1 mg ml^{-1})
Bolus: 0.01 mg kg^{-1}
Add: 1 ml (1:100) to 9 ml NaCl
Administer 0.1 ml kg^{-1} i.v. slowly

Dopamine hydrochloride (4%; 40 mg ml^{-1})
Constant infusion
Rate: 2.0–10.0 μg kg^{-1} min^{-1}
Add: 2 ml (80 mg) to 500 ml 5% dextrose in water to give 160 μg ml^{-1}
Infuse 0.01–0.06 ml kg^{-1} min^{-1}

Dobutamine hydrochloride (1.25%; 12.5 mg ml^{-1})
Constant infusion
Rate: 2.0–15 μg kg^{-1} min^{-1}
Add: 8 ml (100 mg) to 500 ml of 5% dextrose in water to give 200 μg ml^{-1}
Infuse 0.01 ml kg^{-1} min^{-1} to 0.07 ml kg^{-1} min^{-1}.

Atropine sulphate (0.5 mg ml^{-1})
Bolus: 0.02–0.04 mg kg^{-1} i.v.

Glycopyrronium (glycopyrrolate)
Bolus: 0.01 mg kg^{-1} i.v.

INOTROPIC AGENTS

Calcium solutions—calcium chloride and calcium gluconate (Calglucon)

Intravenous infusions of calcium are occasionally used during anaesthesia to reduce the myocardial depressant effects of some inhalant anaesthestics such as halothane, methoxyflurane, enflurane and nitrous oxide (Denlinger *et al.*, 1975). Calcium has also been recommended for use in asystolic cardiac arrest and electromechanical dissociation although retrospective and prospective studies have not demonstrated benefits. In fact, they suggest that this practice may be detrimental (Haskins, 1982; Rinke, 1986). Calcium administration is no longer recommended for cardiac arrest unless hyperkalaemia or hypocalcaemia exists (Rinke, 1986).

Calcium has a primary role in the development of phases 0 and 2 of the action potential in the SA node, AV node and Purkinje fibres and phase 2 of the action potential of ventricular muscle fibres (Adams, 1986). As such, it is essential for cardiac automaticity and intracardiac conduction. It also links myocardial membrane depolarization with muscle contraction and intravenous administration of a calcium salt increases myocardial contractility (Mehmel, Krayenbuehl and Rutishauser, 1970; Bristow *et al.*, 1977). The extent of increase depends upon the initial plasma calcium level. When the plasma calcium level is normal prior to administration of calcium, the improvement in cardiac performance is less than when the initial plasma level is low. Halothane decreases the calcium ion flux through the sarcolemma and disturbs the sarcoplasmic reticular uptake and release of calcium (Lynch, Vogel and Sperelakis, 1981). Intravenous calcium administration may partly counteract this action of halothane. Myocardial oxygen consumption is increased by the administration of calcium salts without augmentation of coronary blood flow but this effect is not as marked as that induced by isoproterenol.

The autonomic nervous system is involved in the peripheral response to calcium administration (Drop, 1985). Calcium stimulates the release of catecholamines from the adrenal medulla and peripheral autonomic nerve endings (Douglas and Rubin, 1963). Hypercalcaemia may also directly stimulate α- and β-adrenoceptors (Douglas and Rubin, 1963). Calcium administration may increase the peripheral vascular resistance, especially when there is no enhancement of the cardiac output to reflexly counteract this effect.

Following an intravenous bolus of calcium, peak plasma levels occur within 3 minutes and then decline over the next 15 minutes.

In the clinical setting, repeated administration of intravenous calcium results in progressively lesser clinical responses.

Calcium toxicity is manifested by sinus dysrhythmias, bradycardia, AV dissociation or junctional rhythms (Lown, Black and Moore, 1960; Carlon *et al.*, 1978). The most consistent ECG change in dogs is elevation of the ST segment. Coronary artery spasm and respiratory failure have been reported in unanaesthetized people who have ben administered clinical doses (Drop, 1985; Kaplan, 1986). Extravasation may cause irritation of the vessel walls and necrosis of subcutaneous tissue.

Amrinone (Inocor), milrinone

Recently, a group of new inotropic agents have been developed for use in human patients with cardiac failure and are of potential benefit in patients with cardiogenic and septic shock. These drugs have yet to be adequately assessed and presently should only be used where all else has failed. With further work, these agents may have a valuable function as intraoperative cardiac support agents and may help overcome some of the myocardial depression induced by most anaesthetic agents. Perhaps the most studied of this group is the bipyridine compound amrinone and its more potent analogue, milrinone (Goldstein, 1986).

The mechanisms of action of amrinone and milrinone are diverse and not entirely clear. The predominant activity is thought to be inhibition of myocardial phosphodiesterase III, which increases cardiac cAMP (Endoh *et al.* 1986). The intracellular calcium levels are also increased and the sensitivity of contractile protein to calcium may be altered (Sutko, Kenyon and Reeves, 1986).

Intravenous amrinone has been demonstrated to increase the cardiac output by 30–69% in patients with heart failure without altering heart rate or blood pressure (Goldstein, 1986). In addition to their positive inotropic activity, amrinone and milrinone cause peripheral and coronary vasodilatation which is independent of reflex autonomic activity (Goldstein, 1986). The fall in arterial blood pressure is sufficient to be of concern at dosages which reverse halothane-induced depression of cardiac output (Boncyk, Redon and Rusy, 1984). A fall in myocardial oxygen consumption has been demonstrated in animals with cardiac dysfunction following amrinone administration despite the rise in cardiac output (Goldstein, 1986).

Electrocardiographically, amrinone decreases the atrial refractory period and AV nodal functional refractory period. AV node conduction is improved. A major advantage of amrinone over the catecholamines is that amrinone does not increase the risk of ventricular tachycardia (Goldstein, 1986).

The maximum effects of amrinone occur 2 minutes after an intravenous bolus and the improvement in cardiac function lasts approximately 60 minutes (Goldstein, 1986). In normal human volunteers, the half-life is 2.6 hours, but it can be up to 5.8 hours in patients with chronic heart failure. Between 10 and 40% of the drug is excreted unchanged in the urine.

To date, very few side effects of amrinone have been reported. Reversible thrombocytopenia has occurred in about 4% of human patients (Goldstein, 1986) and dysrhythmias have occurred following rapid intravenous bolus administration. Bolus administration should be given over a 3-minute period.

CONCLUSION

The approach to pharmacological management of intraoperative cardiovascular disturbances is rapidly changing. Until recently, there have been a limited number of drugs available for use and these were employed on an almost empirical basis. Knowledge of the mechanisms of intraoperative cardiovascular disorders has grown as has information on the pharmacology of cardiovascular support agents. Armed with these facts, a clinician is now permitted to rationally choose a drug for any given condition. For many of the agents discussed, certain pharmacological activities have been well known for a long time, but it is evident that this knowledge is far from complete. Further investigation is required to ensure their appropriate and safe use. Other drugs which are available on an investigational basis only also demand further study to determine their potential value in the management of intraoperative cardiovascular crises in the small animal patient.

ACKNOWLEDGEMENTS

The authors would like to thank Dr P. Kaplan for reviewing the chapter.

REFERENCES

Adams, H. R. (1982). In *Veterinary Pharmacology and Therapeutics*, 5th edn, p. 466. New York: Macmillan Publishing Co. Inc.
Adams, H. R. (1986). *Journal of the American Veterinary Medical Association* **189**, 525.
Anderson, J. L. (1984). *Clinical Therapeutics* **6**, 125.
Atlee, J. L. (1985). *Perioperative Cardiac Dysrhythmias: Mechanisms,*

Recognition and Management, p. 280. Chicago: Year Book Medical Publishers Inc.

Bednarski, R. M. and Muir, W. W. (1983). *American Journal of Veterinary Research* **44**, 2341.

Bigger, J. T. (1980). In *Heart Disease: A Textbook of Cardiovascular Medicine*, p. 691. Philadelphia: W. B. Saunders Co.

Bonagura, J. D. and Muir, W. W. (1985). In *Essentials of Canine and Feline Electrocardiography: Interpretation and Treatment*, 2nd edn, p. 281. Philadelphia: Lea and Febiger.

Boncyk, J., Redon, D. and Rusy, B. (1984). In *Research Communications in Chemical Pathology and Pharmacology* **44**, No. 3.

Bristow, M. R., Schwartz, H. D., Binnetti, G., Harrison, D. C. and Daniels, J. R. (1977). *Circulation Research* **41**, 565.

Carlon, G. C., Howland, W. S., Goldiner, P. S., Kahn, R. C., Bertoni, G. and Turnbull, A. D. (1978). *Archives of Surgery* **113**, 882.

Chelly, J. E., Hysing, E. S., Abernethy, D. R., Doursout, M. and Merin, R. G. (1986a) *Anesthesiology* **65**, 266

Chelly, J. E., Rogers, K., Hysing, E. S., Taylor, A., Hartley, C. and Merlin, R. G. (1986b). *Anesthesiology* **64**, 560.

Chernow, B. and Zolaga, G. P. (1987). *Medical Clinics of North America* **71**, 541.

Chernow, B., Rainery, T. G. and Lake, C. R. (1982). *Critical Care Medicine* **10**, 409.

Chung, D. C. and Laschuck, M. J. (1984). *Canadian Anaesthesiology Society* **31**, 430.

Crowe, D. T. and Calvert, C. A. (1984). In *Veterinary Trauma and Critical Care*, p. 121. Philadelphia: Lea and Febiger.

Davis, L. E. (1984). In *Veterinary Trauma and Critical Care*, p. 287. Philadelphia: Lea and Febiger.

Denlinger, J. K., Kaplan, J. A., Lecky, J. H. and Wollman, H. (1975). *Anesthesiology* **42**, 390.

Dodman, N. H., Seeler, D. C. and Court, M. H. (1984). *British Veterinary Journal* **140**, 505.

Donegan, J. H. (1986). In *Anesthesia*, 2nd edn, p. 2128. New York: Churchill Livingstone.

Douglas, W. W. and Rubin, R. P. (1963). *Journal of Physiology* **167**, 288.

Drop, J. L. (1985). *Anesthesia and Analgesia* **64**, 432.

Endoh, M., Yanagisawa, T., Tairo, N. and Blinks, J. R. (1986). *Circulation* **73**, 111.

Feinberg, B. I., La Mantia, K. and Levy, W. J. (1986). *Anesthesia and Analgesia* **65**, S1–S170.

Goldstein, R. A. (1986). *Circulation* **73**, 111.

Hamlin, R. L., Dutta, S. and Smith, C. R. (1971). *American Journal of Veterinary Research* **32**, 1391.

Haskins, S. C. (1982). *Compendium on Continuing Education* **4**, 170.

Ikeda, M., Dohi, T. and Tsujimoto, A. (1983). *American Society of Anesthesiologists: Refresher Course 38*, 495.

Kaplan, J. A. (1986). In *Anesthesia*, 2 edn, p. 1193. New York: Churchill Livingstone.

Katz, A. M. (1977). In *Physiology of the Heart*, Chapter 19. New York: Raven Press.

Lawson, N. W. and Wallfische, H. K. (1986). *International Anesthesia Research Society Review Course Lectures*, 140.

Lown B., Black, H. and Moore, F. D. (1960). *American Journal of Cardiology* **6**, 309.

Lynch, C., Vogel, S. Sperelakis, N. (1981). *Anesthesiology* **55**, 360.

Maze and Smith (1983) *Anesthesiology* **59**, 322.

Mehmel, H., Krayenbuehl, H. P. and Rutishauser, W. (1970). *Journal of Applied Physiology* **29**, 637.

Merin, R. G. (1981). *Anesthesiology* **55**, 200.

Merin. R. G. (1986). In *Anesthesia*, 2nd edn. p. 976. New York: Churchill Livingstone.

Miller, R. D. and Savarese, J. J. (1986). In *Anesthesia*, 2nd edn, p. 889. New York: Churchill Livingstone.

Mirakhur, R. K. (1979). *Anaesthesia* **34**, 458.

Muir, W. W. (1978). *Journal of the American Veterinary Medical Association* **172**, 192.

Muir, W. W. and Sams, R. (1984). *The Compendium on Continuing Education* **6**, No. 2.

Muir, W. W., Werner, L. L. and Hamlin, R. L. (1975). *American Journal of Veterinary Research* **36**, 1299.

Novotny, M. J. and Adams, H. R. (1986). *Journal of the American Veterinary Medical Association* **189**, 533.

Ogilvie, R. I. (1982). *Canadian Journal of Physiology and Pharmacology* **60**, 968.

Prys-Roberts, C. (1980). In *The Circulation in Anesthesia: Applied Physiology and Pharmacology*, p. 375. London: Blackwell Scientific Publications.

Rinke, C. M. (1986). *Journal of the American Medical Association* **255**, 2992.

Soma, L. R. (1974). In *Textbook of Veterinary Anesthesia*, p. 178. Baltimore: Williams and Wilkins.

Stoelting, R. K. (1987) In *Pharmacology and Physiology in Anesthetic Practice*, p. 233. Philadelphia: J. B. Lippincott Company.

Sutko, J. L., Kenyon, J. L. and Reeves, J. P. (1986). *Circulation* **73**, 111.

Tanaka, K. and Tamasaki, M. (1966). *Nature* **209**, 207.

Tilley, L. P., (1985). In *Essentials of Canine and Feline Electrocardiography: Interpretation and Treatment*, 2nd edn, p. 55. Philadelphia: Lea and Febiger.

Vaughan Williams, E. M. (1984). *Journal of Clinical Pharmacology* **24**, 129.

Wilcke, J. R. (1985). In *Handbook of Small Animal Therapeutics*, p. 276. New York: Churchill Livingstone.

8

Anaesthesia for patients with disease of the hepatic, renal or gastrointestinal systems

The liver, kidneys and gastrointestinal system perform most of the non-volatile excretory functions of the body. Many essential processes depend on normal liver function including metabolism of carbohydrate, fat and protein and inactivation of hormones and drugs. The kidneys and gastrointestinal tract are involved in maintaining the volume and composition of the extracellular fluid. Adequate hepatic and renal function are particularly important from the anaesthetist's viewpoint as many anaesthetic agents are metabolized or excreted by the liver or kidneys.

Disturbances in hepatic, renal and gastrointestinal function increase the risk of general anaesthesia by altering the sensitivity of the patient to anaesthetic agents and by causing derangements in fluid and electrolyte balance. Anaesthetic agents may exacerbate hepatic, renal or gastrointestinal dysfunction, either directly, or indirectly by reducing splanchnic blood supply and oxygen delivery. Deleterious effects on organ function are more likely when such changes are profound or prolonged and accompanied by hypoxaemia.

Identification and accurate assessment of hepatic, renal and gastrointestinal dysfunction are important prior to anaesthesia. Diagnosis is sometimes difficult and some disturbances become evident only after thorough examination of the patient and the use of ancillary diagnostic tests. The formulation of an appropriate anaesthetic regimen should be based on the nature of the disease process and the physical status of the animal at the time of surgery. Appreciation of the physiological changes produced by anaesthesia is also important. The following discussion deals with the selection of anaesthetic techniques suitable for patients with hepatic, renal and gastrointestinal disease.

Table 1. Classification of patients with hepatic dysfunction

Group	Clinical history	Clinical exam	Laboratory tests	ASA risk status
1 (mild)	−	−	+	II
2 (moderate)	(+)	(+)	++	III
3 (severe)	+	++	++	IV or V

HEPATIC DISEASE AND ANAESTHESIA

Preanaesthetic considerations

Patients with hepatic disorders may be classified into three arbitrary groups:

1. patients with *mild* hepatic dysfunction which can only be appreciated when appropriate laboratory tests are performed;
2. patients with *moderate* hypatic dysfunction, tentatively diagnosed by clinical evaluation and subsequently confirmed by laboratory tests; and
3. patients with *severe* hepatic disease which can be diagnosed by clinical examination alone.

The anaesthetic risk to the patient is dependent on the extent of hepatic dysfunction (Table 1).

A typical history of liver dysfunction is often relatively non-specific and may include features such as dullness, listlessness, depression, anorexia, vomition, diarrhoea and weight loss. In patients with severe liver disease, signs of hepatic encephalopathy may be reported. Clinical examination of mildly affected cases may reveal nothing more specific than evidence of a gastrointestinal disorder but advanced cases will present with more typical signs of hepatic disease. These include icterus, cachexia, ascites, neurological disturbances and, in some cases, palpable changes in liver size, shape or consistency (Dodman, Engelking and Anwer, 1987).

Results of laboratory tests which may indicate hepatic dysfunction include: low serum albumin, prolonged blood clotting times, increased serum bilirubin, increased serum activity of alanine aminotransferase, sorbitol dehydrogenase, glutamate dehydrogenase or arginase. It should be appreciated, however, that none of these tests on its own is specific for hepatocellular or biliary tract dysfunction. Consequently, laboratory test results should be interpreted carefully with consideration for the nature and extent of deviations from the normal range. More elaborate tests may be indicated if results are equivocal. Such tests include isoenzyme analysis, bile acid analysis and plasma clearance of dyes which are principally excreted by the liver. Ancillary aids to diagnosis include radiography, positive contrast hepatic angiography and liver biopsy.

Where there is pre-existing liver disease, anaesthesia and surgery may be followed by a severe deterioration in liver function and, on occasion, the development of acute liver failure (Strunin, 1980). If unfavourable reactions to anaesthesia are to be avoided in patients with liver disease it is necessary to:

1. provide appropriate preoperative supportive therapy;
2. avoid drugs which are extensively metabolized or excreted by the liver;
3. avoid agents which are potentially hepatotoxic;
4. maintain hepatic oxygenation by preventing hypoxaemic episodes; and
5. maintain cardiac output and blood pressure to preserve hepatic blood flow and oxygen flux.

Patients with mild hepatic dysfunction require little special preparation prior to anaesthesia. Where clinical signs of disease are evident, however, the condition of the animal should be improved by medical management prior to anaesthesia and surgery (Table 2). This may mean a delay in surgery until the anaesthetic risk to the patient is acceptable. In general, fluid and electrolyte disturbances should be corrected, plasma oncotic pressure should be normalized by the intravenous administration of plasma or dextrans, and blood clotting deficiencies or anaemia should be corrected by transfusion of cross-matched fresh whole blood. If the prothrombin time is prolonged, vitamin K therapy should be instituted before surgery and anaesthesia (Strunin, 1980). Hypoglycaemia, which may be present in massive liver cell necrosis, should be treated by the intravenous administration of 10% dextrose (Cuschieri, 1980). In such cases the blood glucose level should be monitored closely.

It is generally recognized that patients with liver disease have an altered response to anaesthetic agents. Decreased hepatic blood flow, common to some forms of hepatic disease, may prolong the pharmacological action of agents by decreasing hepatic clearance. This effect is more pronounced for drugs with a high hepatic extracton efficiency. Hepatic extraction efficiency, which is dependent on the interaction of drugs and hepatic microsomes, may also be reduced in liver disease with a resultant decrease in hepatic clearance of anaesthetic drugs. When hypoalbuminaemia is present, the bound : unbound ratio will decrease for protein-bound drugs. This can result in a greater peak intensity of

Table 2. Preanaesthetic preparation of patient with hepatic dysfunction

Type of disorder	Example	Preanaesthetic preparation
Congenital	Portocaval shunt (with CNS signs)	Dietary management (decrease protein intake)
Traumatic	Laceration (with haemorrhage)	Treat for haemorrhagic shock
Infectious	Leptospirosis	Treat with antibiotics
Neoplastic	Bile duct carcinoma	None (consider prognosis)
Hormonal	Fatty liver (secondary to diabetes mellitus)	Treat primary (hormonal) disturbance
Metabolic	Copper storage disease with accompanying gastrointestinal disturbance	Establish appropriate fluid therapy
Toxic	Acute: ingestion of hepatotoxin	Gastric lavage or forced emesis
	Chronic: cirrhosis (with ascites)	Drain ascitic fluid (consider prognosis)

pharmacological action particularly for highly protein-bound drugs (Dundee and McCaughey, 1980). Several drugs have been shown to exhibit decreased binding and an increased volume of distribution in liver disease (Sear, 1984). In chronic liver failure, an increase in the number of central gamma-aminobutyric acid (GABA) receptors has been postulated to account for the enhanced response of these patients to GABA-mimetic agents such as benzodiazepines and barbiturates (Jones *et al.*, 1985).

Premedication

Phenothiazine tranquillizers may have a profound effect in patients with liver dysfunction and should be employed cautiously in such cases. Acepromazine is not hepatotoxic, but chlorpromazine, a closely related compound, has been reported to cause cholestatic jaundice in man after a single administration (Zarowitz and Friedman, 1957). Chlorpromazine has also been reported to decrease splanchnic blood flow (Kelman, 1969). Phenothiazines, in general, may have other adverse effects mediated indirectly via their hypothermic action (Pugh, 1964). Another potential problem in patients with hepatic encephalopathy is that phenothiazines may lower the ictal threshold and precipitate seizures. After consideration of the available data it appears that phenothiazines should be reserved for patients with mild disease and even then only after due consideration of possible adverse sequelae.

Xylazine is particularly unsuitable for use in patients with liver disease because of the profound physiological depression it causes (Klide, Calderwood and Soma, 1975; Biewenga *et al.*, 1978; Kolata and Rawlings, 1982). Even moderate doses of xylazine have been reported to cause a significant fall in arterial oxygen tension and cardiac output in dogs (McDonnell and Van Gorder, 1982). In one recent study, Haskins, Patz and Farver (1986) concluded that xylazine should not be used in dogs with visceral organ insufficiency because of evidence of reduced oxygen delivery to the tissues. The present authors concur with this opinion and prefer to avoid xylazine in all such patients. Similar considerations apply to the use of medetomidine in animals with hepatic disease since this drug has an almost identical pharmacodynamic profile to xylazine.

Diazepam may be the most appropriate sedative for animals with liver disease. Although it does not exhibit a tranquillizing effect in normal dogs and may even cause restlessness or excitement, this agent does seem to have a sedative effect in patients that become obtund as a result of central nervous system disease or metabolic disorders (Haskins, Farver and Patz, 1986). A major advantage of diazepam is that it is said to produce minimal cardiopulmonary disturbance (Haskins, Farver and Patz, 1986; Jones, Stehling and Zauder, 1979). Despite this apparent safety factor, diazepam should be used cautiously when there is severe liver disease because it may precipitate respiratory failure in this situation (Cuschieri, 1980). It is also noteworthy that cholestatic jaundice has been reported following diazepam administration in man (Read, 1979). Finally, increased cerebral sensitivity to diazepam coupled with slowed biotransformation may result in a delayed recovery from anaesthesia in some patients with liver disease (Branch *et al.*, 1976).

Opioid analgesic drugs are probably safer than tranquillizers or sedatives for premedication of patients with hepatic disease. Several studies indicate that these agents have little or no adverse effect on the liver (Zimmerman, 1978; White, 1984). Another advantage of opioid agents is that their effects can be rapidly reversed with a specific antagonist should this become necessary. It should be remembered that opioid drugs may cause ventilatory depression in animals (Benson *et al.*, 1987; Carter and Mercer, 1987; Haskins *et al.*, 1987) and the minimum effective dose should be used. Opioid analgesic drugs increase tone in the sphincter of Oddi and may be unsuitable when there is biliary retention. These agents also cause bradycardia in dogs (Benson *et al.*, 1987) and an anticholinergic agent such as atropine or glycopyrrolate should be administered concomitantly (Dodman, Seeler and Court, 1984). Anticholinergic agents are relatively safe for use in patients with hepatic disease. Their pharmacological action may be prolonged when there is hepatic dysfunction, although this is usually of little consequence to a patient.

In severely debilitated patients, it may be best to avoid sedative premedication.

Induction of anaesthesia

Preoxygenation of patients with liver disease for 2–3 minutes prior to the induction of general anaesthesia is recommended to prevent hypoxaemia. Subsequently, anaesthesia may be induced by the administration of an intravenous or inhalational anaesthetic agent.

Thiobarbiturates are satisfactory for intravenous induction of anaesthesia in patients with mild to moderate liver disease but should be used sparingly, if at all, when hepatic disease is severe. Hall and Clarke (1983) report a prolongation of the action of thiopentone in experimental animals following liver damage by other agents. They conclude that hepatic detoxication plays a significant role in recovery from thiopentone. Recently, it has been demonstrated that prolonged recovery from the effects of thiopentone in greyhounds is probably caused by a deficiency in intrinsic hepatic metabolism (Ilkiw, Sampson and Cutler, 1985; Sams and Muir, 1986). This is further evidence in support of the contention that hepatic metabolism is a major factor in recovery from thiobarbiturate anaesthesia. If thiobarbiturates are to be used in patients with liver disease they should be administered cautiously using the minimum effective dose.

Methohexitone may be a more logical choice in patients with hepatic dysfunction as the marked fat solubility of this drug coupled with more rapid hepatic metabolism will result in a faster recovery than occurs with thiopentone (Hall and Clarke, 1983). Minimal doses should be used and measures should be taken to prevent excitement and muscle tremors characteristic of this agent (Hall and Clarke, 1983). Methohexitone should be used extremely cautiously in patients with severe hepatic disease because altered cerebral sensitivity and decreased protein binding may result in unpredictably profound narcosis and physiological depression.

Ketamine may be used for induction of anaesthesia in cats with mild or moderate hepatic dysfunction. In severe liver disease, caveats similar to those which apply when using thiobarbiturates are pertinent. Decreased cardiac and pulmonary performance and reduced peripheral oxygen transport have been reported in critically ill human patients following intravenous administration of ketamine (Waxman, Shoemaker and Lippmann, 1980). Ketamine should be administered slowly intravenously and to effect when used for induction of anaesthesia in debilitated cats. In this species, 87% of an administered dose of ketamine is excreted unchanged in the urine therefore recovery from its effects is not dependent on hepatic metabolism (Lumb and Jones, 1984). Ketamine has been described for induction of anaesthesia in dogs either alone (Haskins, Farver and Patz, 1985), or following diazepam or xylazine pretreatment (Haskins, Farver and Patz, 1986; Haskins, Patz and Farver, 1986). The present authors contend, however, that the use of ketamine alone in dogs cannot be condoned because of the potential for overt seizure activity and exuberant spontaneous movement (Stephenson, Blevins and Christie, 1978; Haskins, Farver and Patz, 1985). Xylazine pretreatment, a frequent adjunct to ketamine anaesthesia, is undesirable in patients with liver disease for reasons previously discussed. The use of diazepam with ketamine may be a more reasonable combination for induction of anaesthesia in dogs wth mild to moderate hepatic disease as some of the unpleasant side effects of ketamine such as muscle hypertonus and seizure activity are reduced without significant additional physiological depression (Haskins, Farver and Patz, 1986). Offset against this, vomition may be encountered more frequently when a diazepam–ketamine combination is used for induction of anaesthesia than when ketamine is used alone (Haskins, Farver and Patz, 1986). In dogs, the half-life of ketamine may be prolonged when hepatic disease is severe.

Induction of anaesthesia in cats with liver disease using the steroid anaesthetic mixture alphaxalone–alphadolone acetate (Saffan, Glaxo Laboratories Ltd, Middlesex) is probably as safe as any method of intravenous induction. The mixture has a high safety margin when compared to thiopentone or ketamine in cats (Child *et al.*, 1972a) and is rapidly metabolized by the liver as well as being excreted in the urine in appreciable amounts (Card, McCulloch and Pratt, 1972; Child *et al.*, 1972b). Alphaxalone-alphadolone acetate should not be given to dogs, however, because of the potential for massive histamine release (Davis and Pearce, 1972).

Induction of narcosis in dogs with liver disease by the intravenous administration of opioid agents may be the safest and most appropriate injectable anaesthetic technique. Oxymorphone will sometimes produce chemical restraint and narcosis which is sufficient to permit orotracheal intubation. The technique of administration has been described by Sawyer (1982). Other opioid drugs, such as pethidine, fentanyl, sufentanyl and butorphanol, have also been used, either alone or following sedative premedication for the intravenous induction of narcosis in dogs (Sawyer, 1982;

Erhardt *et al.*, 1986; Benson *et al.*, 1987). Precautions should be taken to prevent hypoxaemia secondary to ventilatory depression when large doses of opioid agents are employed for this purpose (Sawyer, 1982).

Most of the currently used volatile anaesthetic agents are satisfactory for inhalational induction of anaesthesia in patients with liver disease. Isoflurane is the most appropriate choice, since it has a low blood gas solubility and therefore induction is rapid. This agent is also minimally metabolized by the liver (Eger, 1984). The recommended technique is to increase the concentration of anaesthetic slowly in stepwise fashion until anaesthetic induction is complete. This will minimize excitement of the patient during induction. Inhalational induction is probably the safest technique in patients with hepatic disease and should be employed if there is any uncertainty regarding the safety of other methods. If nitrous oxide is used along with a volatile agent to facilitate anaesthetic induction in a debilitated patient, it should not be used at a concentration greater than 50% in oxygen to reduce the potential for hypoxaemia.

Maintenance of anaesthesia

Anaesthesia should be maintained with a volatile anaesthetic. These agents are primarily excreted through the lungs and do not rely on hepatic metabolism to terminate their action. Isoflurane is the inhalational anaesthetic agent of choice although halothane may also be used with reasonable safety. Halothane is not directly hepatotoxic but there is evidence that, under certain circumstances, it can be metabolized to free radicals which are toxic to the liver (Brown, 1972; Cousins, 1984). To date this has been the most viable explanation for halothane-associated hepatitis, which is a rare but well-recognized clinical entity in human anaesthetic practice. Recent experimental studies indicate that a prominent reduction in liver blood flow and associated hepatic oxygen deprivation may also be partly responsible for halothane-associated hepatic damage (Baden *et al.*, 1987; Hursh, Gelman and Bradley, 1987). The relative merits of isoflurane, halothane, methoxyflurane and nitrous oxide for maintenance of anaesthesia in patients with liver disease are discussed in detail elsewhere (Dodman, Engleking and Anwer, 1987).

When a skilled anaesthetist is available, balanced anaesthetic techniques provide a greater safety margin for patients with moderate to severe hepatic dysfunction. In balanced anaesthesia, ventilation is controlled and muscle relaxation and somatic reflex suppression are supplied independently by means of a neuromuscular blocking agent (Hart, 1971). Atracurium is the relaxant of choice since it does not rely on normal hepatic function to terminate its action. This agent is broken down in plasma by a temperature and pH-dependent reaction called Hoffman elimination (Klein, 1987). Vecuronium, another relatively new relaxant, relies on both hepatic and renal elimination processes (Lebrault *et al.*, 1985). The elimination half-life and duration of action of vecuronium were shown to be prolonged in human patients with cirrhosis, but these alterations were relatively modest (Duvaldstein *et al.*, 1983). Although pancuronium is primarily excreted through the kidneys, the elimination half-life of this relaxant was reported to be increased by 100% in human patients with cirrhosis or cholestasis, possibly as a result of an increase in the volume of distribution of the drug (Duvaldstein *et al.*, 1983).

During maintenance of anaesthesia it is important to monitor the patient adequately and to maintain the body temperature and fluid status (Dodman, Seeler and Court, 1984). When muscle relaxants are employed the degree and duration of neuromuscular blockade should be monitored closely (Ali, 1985). In severely ill patients serial measurements of arterial blood pressure, arterial blood gases and blood glucose level will provide valuable information.

Recovery

Patients should be allowed to recover from anaesthesia in a warm, well-lit area and should receive constant surveillance until they are fully recovered (Dodman, Seeler and Court, 1984). Oxygen supplementation and fluid administration are often required during this period and postoperative analgesia should be supplied when necessary (Dodman, Seeler and Court, 1984).

RENAL DISEASE AND ANAESTHESIA

Preanaesthetic considerations

Small animal patients with renal disease often require general anaesthesia for surgical or medical procedures. The majority of these patients present with varying degrees of physiologically compensated renal dysfunction. Occasionally, it may be necessary to anaesthetize a patient in renal failure. The degree of renal dysfunction determines the magnitude of the physiological disturbance encountered and subsequently anaesthetic risk to the patient. Derangements in renal function commonly result in altered fluid and electrolyte balance and acid-base disturbances. Preoperative assessment of patients with azotaemia should be

Table 3. Use of laboratory data to differentiate between prerenal, postrenal and renal causes of renal failure

Laboratory test	Aetiology of azotaemia		
	Prerenal	Renal	Postrenal
Urea levels	1+	1–3+	1–3+
Creatinine levels	1+	1–3+	1–3+
Urine specific gravity*	> 1.030†	< 1.030†	Variable
	> 1.035‡	< 1.035‡	
Urine output	Decreased	Variable	Anuria or oliguiria

* Prior to fluid administration.
† Canine.
‡Feline.
Note: 1+ means slight elevation of laboratory values over normal; 1–3+ means slight to moderate elevation.

based on clinical history, physical examination and analysis of laboratory data (Table 3). Routine laboratory tests, though relatively non-specific, will at least give some indication of the severity of the condition and will provide a baseline for estimating the response to therapy (Grauer, 1985; Benson and Thurmon, 1987). More specific tests are indicated to distinguish the various forms of renal disease which may be present (Lewis, 1963). An overview of these tests and their interpretation has been presented by Osborne and Polzin (1983a,b).

Once the risk of anaesthesia has been determined, the clinician should ensure appropriate preoperative preparation of the patient. One to two hours of water deprivation is normally adequate to prevent vomition in small animal patients (Dodman, Seeler and Court, 1984). Prolonged fluid restriction is contraindicated in patients with impaired renal concentrating ability as it may precipitate a uraemic crisis (Hall and Clarke, 1983). Uraemia should be avoided as it increases the sensitivity of the patient to anaesthetic agents. This increased sensitivity is not directly caused by the elevation in blood urea concentration, but is related to associated changes of dehydration, electrolyte imbalance, and acid–base disturbance. In situations where prolonged water deprivation is unavoidable, the fluid status of the animal should be maintained by preoperative administration of intravenous fluids.

Fluid therapy is the mainstay of therapy when renal dysfunction is present. In patients that are uraemic, polyionic electrolyte solutions, such as lactated Ringer's soluion, should be administered intravenously. Rehydration of the uraemic patient will increase renal perfusion and improve renal function. This is usually all that is necessary for patients with prerenal uraemia resulting from dehydration. Small animal patients with postrenal obstructive disease also benefit from rehydration, but these patients, and animals which present in acute renal failure, require specific treatment in addition to supportive therapy (Burrows and Bovee, 1978; Dibartola, 1980). Patients that are anaemic (haematocrit <20%) or hypoproteinaemic (total serum protein <3.5 g dl^{-1}) as a result of chronic renal disease may require transfusion with cross-matched fresh whole blood or plasma prior to anaesthesia.

When severe renal dysfunction is evident, the clinician should anticipate acid–base and electrolyte disturbances. Metabolic acidosis is probably the most common acid–base disturbance in patients with renal disease. Mild to moderate acidosis will usually respond to intravenous therapy with a solution containing a bicarbonate precursor, such as lactate or acetate. Sodium bicarbonate is indicated in patients with severe metabolic acidosis. Blood gas analysis is the definitive method for the diagnosis and monitoring of acid–base disturbances. When blood gas analysis is not available, bicarbonate deficits may be estimated and treated empirically (Seeler and Thurmon, 1985).

Disturbances in serum potassium level often accompany acid–base imbalance. Hyperkalaemia occurs in association with acidosis in patients with renal disease. The serum potassium concentration increases by 0.6 mEq l^{-1} for each 0.1 pH unit decrease in pH (Seeler and Thurmon, 1985). Small animal patients whose serum potassium is above 6.0 mEq l^{-1} should not be anaesthetized for elective procedures.

Hyperkalaemia can be treated by the intravenous administration of potassium-free solutions such as normal saline or 5% dextrose in water. The serum potassium concentration should be monitored closely since aggressive therapy may cause hypokalaemia (Burrows and Bovee, 1978; Seeler and Thurmon, 1985). The electrocardiogram can be used to estimate serum potassium when immediate analysis of blood samples is not possible. Bradycardia occurs when the serum potassium level is above 6.5 mEq l^{-1}. When the concentration is between 7.0 and 8.0 mEq l^{-1}, tall, peaked T waves become evident. Serum levels in excess of 8.0 mEq l^{-1} result in a decreased PR interval, the disappearance of the P wave and widening of the QRS complex (Seeler and Thurmon, 1985). Cardiac arrest is likely to occur when the serum potassium concentration reaches 9–10 mEq l^{-1}. In critical situations, calcium solutions may be used to antagonize the deleterious cardiac effects of hyperkalaemia. Insulin–dextrose combinations and sodium bicarbonate should be used to rapidly reduce the serum potassium level (Polzin and Osborne, 1985; Seeler and Thurmon, 1985).

Systemic disturbances associated with renal disease affect the pharmacological action of commonly used anaesthetic agents both directly and indirectly. Cerebral depression, which is often present in uraemic patients, will reduce the dose requirement for all central nervous system depressant drugs. Hypoalbuminaemia, associated with protein-losing nephropathies, will also increase sensitivity to protein-bound anaesthetic drugs. This increased sensitivity results from an increase in the proportion of unbound drug available for diffusion into the central nervous system. In human patients with uraemia it has been demonstrated that 56% of thiopentone is unbound compared to 28% in normal subjects (Ghoneim and Pandya, 1975). Metabolic acidosis increases the un-ionized portion of drugs which are weak acids. The pharmacological action of thiobarbiturates is intensified by this mechanism and allowances must be made for this when acidosis is present. Drugs or drugs with active metabolites which are dependent on renal excretion should be used with caution, if at all, in patients with renal dysfunction (Bastron, 1986).

Another consideration when anaesthestizing patients with renal disease is the effect of anaesthetic agents and techniques on renal function. The direct effects of anaesthetic agents on renal function are of minor importance compared with the indirect effects of anaesthesia and surgery. Anaesthesia causes reductions in renal perfusion, urine flow and urine osmolality. These changes are a result of antidiuretic hormone release, sympathetic nervous system activation and increased angiotensin activity. Antidiuretic hormone is released by anaesthetic agents, surgical stimulation and intermittent positive pressure ventilation (Fewell and Bond, 1980; Berry, 1981). When there is an inadequate plane of anaesthesia, surgical stimulation causes excessive release of catecholamines and renin. Increases in sympathoadrenal activity will result in renal vasoconstriction and redirection of renal blood flow from the renal cortex to the medulla with an overall reduction in renal perfusion. Subsequent activation of the renin–angiotensin–aldosterone system may then cause further renal vasoconstriction (Priano, 1984). Good anaesthetic technique is essential to minimize the neurohumoral response to anaesthesia and subsequent adverse renal sequelae. In this context it is important to maintain an adequate depth of anaesthesia and to avoid factors such as hypoxaemia, hypercapnia and hypovolaemia.

Premedication

The objective of premedication is to tranquillize or sedate the dog or cat in order to ensure a smooth induction and maintenance of anaesthesia and to facilitate a peaceful recovery. Reducing stress associated with anaesthesia will minimize potentially adverse effects of sympathetic nervous activation on renal haemodynamics.

Phenothiazines and butyrophenones are suitable for premedication of patients with mild to moderate renal disease and have the advantage of producing mild, long-lasting sedation. These agents, by virtue of their α-adrenergic blocking activity, will decrease arterial pressure and may increase renal blood flow (Bastron and Deutsch, 1976). The latter effect may be beneficial in some forms of renal disease provided the patient is haemodynamically stable. Hypotension or hypovolaemia secondary to severe renal disease are contraindications to the use of these agents.

Opioid analgesic agents may be used to premedicate patients with renal disease. Although large doses of morphine have been shown to increase the release of antidiuretic hormone for up to 24 hours postoperatively in the dog (Bidwai *et al.*, 1975), the significance of this effect in patients with renal disease is unknown. On the other hand, opioid agents have been recommended for use in some patients with renal disease for reasons of cardiovascular and renal haemodynamic stability (Dixon *et al.*, 1970; Bastron and Deutsch, 1976). If opioid agents are employed in anuric patients, their action may be prolonged (Don, Dieppa and Taylor, 1975). In this event, an opioid antagonist such as naloxone may be useful.

In severely depressed patients with renal disease, sedative premedication may not be required. Under these circumstances, the central nervous depressant action of sedative premedication and the pharmacological and physiological sequelae of such treatment may have adverse consequences for the patient. Anticholinergic premedication is relatively safe and may be required in some cases. It has been recommended that atropine should be administered to severely uraemic human patients because they are susceptible to vagal-induced bradycardia and cardiac arrest (Lunding, 1965; Deutsch, 1973).

Induction

Induction techniques vary from the careful intravenous administration of a thiobarbiturate to the use of volatile agents such as halothane or isoflurane. Barbiturates should probably be reserved for use in mild cases of renal disease as their physiologically depressant actions will be exaggerated in moderate to severe renal dysfunction. A reduction in dose requirement of barbiturate should always be anticipated in renal disease and these agents should be administered slowly and to effect in this situation. Features of renal disease which increase the sensitivity of patients to the effects of thiobarbiturates include hypotension, hypovolaemia, dehydration, acidosis and hypoalbuminaemia. Pre-existing haemodynamic albuminaemia and acidosis together increase the proportion of unbound, un-ionized drug causing a more profound effect from a given dose.

The use of opioid agents to induce narcosis and facilitate orotracheal intubation of the patient is a relatively safe induction technique in dogs with renal disease. A number of opioid drugs and neuroleptanalgesic combinations have been used for induction of narcosis in dogs as referenced in an earlier section. The neuroleptanalgesic combination of fentanyl and droperidol has been reported to have minimal adverse effects on renal haemodynamics in the dog and in man and may have advantages over other techniques (Gorman and Craythorne, 1966; Bastron and Deutsch, 1976).

Halothane or isoflurane may be used for induction of anaesthesia in patients with renal disease. Methoxyflurane and enflurane should be avoided in high risk situations (Sladen 1982). Inhalational induction, which involves a graded and rapidly reversible administration of the anaesthetic agent, has much to recommend it in terms of patient safety. Provided that the patient does not become excited during inhalational induction, there should be no adverse effects on renal perfusion or renal function.

Maintenance

General anaesthesia should be maintained with a volatile anaesthetic agent delivered in oxygen or oxygen/nitrous oxide mixture. Either halothane or isoflurane are suitable agents although isoflurane has a number of properties which make it the agent of choice in the critically ill animal (Eger, 1981). Minimum effective doses of the inhalant anaesthetics should be employed in physiologically depressed patients in order to reduce anaesthetic-induced cardiopulmonary depression and preserve renal blood flow. Methoxyflurane should be avoided for maintenance of anaesthesia in patients with renal disease. This agent is extensively biotransformed by the liver and its metabolites have been demonstrated to possess nephrotoxic properties in man (Benson and Brock, 1980; Mazze, 1984). Free fluoride ions appear to be implicated in methoxyflurane-related nephrotoxicity (Benson and Thurmon, 1987). In the dog, increased serum fluoride concentration and transient clinical signs of nephropathy have been reported to follow methoxyflurane anaesthesia (Pedersoli, 1977). Although dogs may be more resistant to the effects of fluoride ions (Benson and Thurmon, 1987), it is prudent to avoid a potentially nephrotoxic agent when a nephropathy exists.

Balanced anaesthetic techniques using nitrous oxide and muscle relaxants in combination with inhalant anaesthetics are useful in critically ill patients. Nitrous oxide reduces the requirement of the more physiologically depressant volatile anaesthetic agent and also provides background analgesia. The muscle relaxants of choice for patients with renal disease are vecuronium and atracurium. Neither of these agents relies on renal excretion to terminate its action (Klein, 1987). Pancuronium and gallamine should be avoided as their action is prolonged when renal dysfunction is present (Miller, 1983; Klein, 1987).

Positive pressure ventilation of the lungs is an essential component of any balanced technique. If properly applied, it is relatively harmless to the patient, but inappropriate application may result in cardiovascular depression, acid-base disturbances and the release of antidiuretic hormone (Fewell and Bond, 1980). Detailed descriptions of balanced anaesthetic techniques are provided in standard veterinary anaesthesia texts (Hall and Clarke, 1983; Short, 1987).

In patients with renal disease, it is important to monitor cardiovascular function, renal function, acid–base status, and serum electrolyte levels. In order to monitor cardiovascular function adequately it is important to measure arterial pressure. This can be accomplished using either direct or indirect blood pressure monitoring equipment. When the mean systemic arterial pressure decreases to less than 70 mmHg, glomerular filtration is reduced and urine production diminishes (Trim, 1979). Renal perfusion can be assessed by monitoring urine output using a Foley catheter and collection chamber. Normal urine production is approximaely 1–2 ml kg^{-1} h^{-1}. If urine output falls below 0.5 ml kg^{-1} h^{-1} renal perfusion may become inadequate.

Intravenous administration of fluids plays a key role in the intraoperative management of patients with renal disease. It is particularly important to attempt to maintain normovolaemia, normotension and adequate renal perfusion in these patients. The recommended intraoperative infusion rate for crystalloid solutions (5–10 ml kg^{-1} h^{-1}) may need to be exceeded in these patients in order to achieve these goals. Blood loss should be replaced as it occurs on a volume-for-volume basis using a colloidal solution or by administering three times the volume of blood lost during a crystalloid solution. Correction of ongoing acid–base or electrolyte abnormalities should continue throughout the anaesthetic procedure and into the recovery period.

Recovery

Monitoring should continue into the recovery period for as long as necessary to ensure that renal function is adequate. Critically ill patients will require more extensive monitoring. It is just as important to maintain the patient's haemodynamic status and fluid balance during the recovery period as it is during the anaesthetic period itself. In severe cases of renal disease, it may be necessary to monitor arterial pressure or central venous pressure and urine output so that intravenous fluids can be titrated accurately to achieve a measured response. Other considerations for recovery of these patients, including the provision of oxygen, heat and analgesia, are similar to those for any seriously debilitated patient (Dodman, Seeler and Court, 1984; Dodman *et al.*, 1987).

GASTROINTESTINAL DISEASE AND ANAESTHESIA

Preanaesthetic considerations

Patients with gastrointestinal tract disease present with a variety of pathophysiological disturbances the nature and extent of which depend on the aetiology and duration of the condition. Fluid and electrolyte imbalance, hypovolaemia and acid–base disturbances are common problems. Cardiac dysrhythmias, mechanical impairment of cardiorespiratory function, endotoxaemia and aspiration pneumonia may also be encountered in some cases. Table 4 lists some of the causes of gastrointestinal disturbances and the typical pathophysiological changes which are associated with them.

Fluid imbalance is important to the anaesthetist because of its adverse effects on the patient's circulatory status. Methods of estimating body deficits have been described elsewhere (Raffe, 1987). Patients in which there had been excessive loss of body fluids as a result of vomition, diarrhoea or gastrointestinal sequestration may present in peripheral circulatory failure. The classical signs of hypovolaemic shock are usually evident in such cases. When clinical signs indicate that peripheral circulatory failure exists, the physiological lesion should be quantitated by measurement of the arterial pressure, central venous pressure and core-to-periphery temperature gradient (Ledingham and Routh, 1979). Restoration of blood volume may be accomplished using crystalloid or colloid solutions. Both methods have their protagonists and under many circumstances either is acceptable (Shoemaker and Hauser, 1979). Colloid solutions such as plasma and dextrans should be used in preference to crystalloids when the plasma protein level is below 3.5 g dl^{-1}.

Septic shock may complicate the clinical picture if the intestinal mucosa becomes ischaemic and the integrity of the blood–gut barrier is lost. In this situation endotoxins will be absorbed from the gastrointestinal tract into the circulation. Endotoxaemia may initially give rise to hyperdynamic shock, a condition in which the cardiac output is temporarily increased (Pascoe, 1987). In such

Table 4. The pathophysiology and clinical signs of some gastrointestinal disorders

Disease	Clinical signs	Pathophysiology
Pyloric stenosis	Projectile vomiting	Loss of chloride-rich gastric secretions causing alkalosis. Loss of sodium, potassium, and water lead to hyponatraemia, hypokalaemia and dehydration
Gastric dilatation volvulus syndrome	Gastric tympany Prostration Circulatory failure	Cardiorespiratory compromise caused by dilated viscus. Peripheral circulatory failure lead to endotoxaemia
Gastritis/gastric foreign body	Frequent vomiting	Similar to that outlined for pyloric stenosis but more severe alkalosis at first. Acidosis latterly
Intestinal lymphosarcoma	Vomition Weight loss Dehydration	Chronic loss of gastrointestinal secretions. Metabolic changes depend on location of lesion. Frequently acidosis and hypokalaemia
Intestinal obstruction (foreign body)	Vomition Hypovolaemia	Acute loss of gastrointestinal secretions (including pancreatic secretions). Acidosis develops early. Occasionally compensatory hyperventilation
Enteritis	Diarrhoea and/or vomiting	Loss of gastrointestinal secretions. Dehydration, hyponatraemia and hypokalaemia may all be present. Acidosis may be present.

cases the mucous membranes may be cherry red, rather than blanched as might be anticipated. Patients in septic shock should be treated with broad spectrum antibiotics prior to surgery. The value of high dose corticosteroid therapy in septic shock is controversial, although recent studies conclude that such treatment is of no benefit (Sprung *et al.*, 1984; Bone *et al.*, 1987; Hinshaw *et al.*,

1987). Flunixin meglumine, a cyclo-oxygenase inhibitor, has been advocated for use in patients with sepsis and has been shown to improve survival in dogs with septic peritonitis (Hardie and Rawlings, 1983; Hardie, Rawlings and Collins, 1985). Narcotic antagonists may also be of value in septic shock because of their beneficial haemodynamic effects (Peters *et al.*, 1981; Groeger, Carlon and Howland, 1983).

Acid–base and electrolyte disturbances are often associated with fluid imbalance resulting from gastrointestinal disease. These disorders are difficult to assess clinically but may be associated with either cardiovascular or respiratory signs. The acid–base and electrolyte changes commonly encountered and accompanying clinical signs are indicated in Table 4. Arterial blood gas analysis and serum chemistry will confirm and quantify suspected metabolic disturbance and electrolyte imbalance. Electrolyte imbalance normally responds to intravenous therapy with a polyionic replacement solution. Lactated Ringer's solution is often adequate for this purpose and has been termed 'the universal replacement solution' (Clark, 1980). Lactated Ringer's solution may be safely administered to critical patients at rates of up to 80 ml kg^{-1} h^{-1} if cardiac and renal function are normal (Pascoe, 1987). The cardiovascular and renal systems maintain the extracellular environment by directly regulating the amount and composition of urine. The kidneys selectively retain only what is needed for restoration and maintenance of homeostasis, provided sufficient quantities of fluid and electrolytes are available. Unfortunately renal concentrating ability may be impaired following severe dehydration and azotaemia. In such cases it is important to treat hyponatraemia aggressively (Tyler *et al.*, 1987). Hypokalaemia should be treated using potassium-supplemented intravenous fluids. Although the serum potassium level can be adjusted reasonably rapidly, repletion of total body potassium may take several days. Acid–base disturbances often correct themselves as fluid and electrolyte balance is restored. The lactate component of lactated Ringer's solution is a precursor of bicarbonate and will assist in the treatment of moderate metabolic acidosis. The conversion of lactate to bicarbonate takes place in the liver in 2–6 hours (Clark, 1980). In severe acidosis, when a more immediate effect is required, it may be necessary to administer sodium bicarbonate. Alkalosis normally responds to intravenous therapy with normal sodium chloride solution.

Cardiac dysrhythmias may occur in association with electrolyte disturbances or may result from myocardial ischaemia or autonomic imbalance. Dysrhythmias are often associated with gastric dilatation volvulus (GDV) syndrome in dogs. These dysrhythmias may be present at the time of the initial examination but may not appear until up to 36 hours later (Muir, 1982). When ventricular premature depolarizations or ventricular tachycardia are present, therapy with intravenously administered lignocaine or procainamide should be initiated preoperatively. Details regarding the treatment of dysrhythmias have been described by Seeler *et al.* (1987).

Mechanical impairment of cardiorespiratory function may occur when the intra-abdominal pressure is elevated as a result of gastrointestinal distension with gas or fluids. This may occur in intestinal obstruction or, more dramatically, in gastric dilatation volvulus syndrome. In the gastric dilatation volvulus syndrome, as the intragastric pressure increases, the gastric circulation, caudal vena cava blood flow and portal venous flow are obstructed. Venous return to the heart and cardiac output are subsequently reduced. In an experimental study in dogs a 64% reduction in cardiac output occurred when the intragastric pressure was increased to 30 mmHg (Orton and Muir, 1983). When gastric distension is severe, intra-abdominal pressure should be relieved preoperatively by stomach tube, paracentesis or gastrostomy.

Aspiration pneumonia is a possible sequel to vomition in small animals that are severely depressed or comatose. This condition is normally treated with broad spectrum antibiotics. Corticosteroid therapy has also been advocated (Lumb and Jones, 1984). Although neither treatment is harmful, the use of prophylactic antibiotics cannot be shown to alter the course of the disease and evidence from animal studies suggests that corticosteroids are ineffective in this situation (Chapman *et al.*, 1974; Spence, 1980). When arterial oxygenation is impaired, supplementary oxygen should be administered preoperatively using a face mask, nasal insufflation, or by means of an oxygen tent or cage. Details of the techniques involved have been described by Court, Dodman and Seeler (1985).

Premedication

The choice of premedicant depends largely on the temperament and physiological status of the patient prior to anaesthesia. When physiological changes are minimal, for example, in cases with mild chronic diarrhoea, no real deviation from standard anaesthetic practice is necessary and the premedicant may be selected to suit the temperament of the animal (Dodman, Seeler and Court, 1984). At the other extreme, a severe case of GDV in the dog may require little or no sedative premedication.

Acepromazine is satisfactory for premedication of most patients with gastrointestinal disease providing central nervous system depression and cardiovascular depression are minimal. In hypovolaemia, a precipitous fall in arterial pressure may occur (Hall and Clarke, 1983), making this agent unsuitable for use in this situation. The antiemetic properties of acepromazine and its spasmolytic effect on smooth muscle may be beneficial in some cases. It should be remembered, however, that acepromazine may increase the likelihood of passive reflux of stomach contents by reducing tone in the gastro-oesophageal sphincter (Strombeck and Harrold, 1985).

Premedication with xylazine is inadvisable in most patients with gastrointestinal disease because it causes profound cardiovascular depression and emesis (Knight, 1980; Lumb and Jones, 1984). Xylazine also causes complete gastrointestinal atony which may enhance the accumulation of intestinal gases. This side effect makes it unsuitable when the gastric or intestinal intraluminal pressure is elevated (Lumb and Jones, 1984). Similar caveats apply to the use of medetomidine in patients with gastrointestinal disease.

Diazepam may be used safely in patients debilitated by gastrointestinal disease as it causes minimal physiological depression. It is reported to reduce the dose of induction and maintenance agents, provide muscle relaxation, and suppress excitatory phenomena encountered when methohexitone is used for induction (Sawyer, 1982; Hall and Clarke, 1983). Unfortunately, diazepam administered alone produces, at best, only mild sedation and, paradoxically, will induce apparent anxiety with increased awareness and restlessness in many animals. This type of response limits the usefulness of this drug in small animals. A more reliable response may be obtained if diazepam is used in combination with an opioid analgesic agent.

Opioid drugs, such as morphine and pethidine, may be used alone or in combination with sedative agents for premedication of small animals with gastrointestinal disease. Morphine stimulates the chemoreceptor trigger zone and frequently causes vomition in dogs (Hall and Clarke, 1983). In addition, morphine has been shown to augment propulsive activity in the ileum and jejunum followed by a period of high tonus with marked and prolonged slowing or arrest of propulsion (Sollmann, 1948). These actions may make morphine unsuitable in some patients. In contrast to morphine, pethidine is less likely to cause vomition and is reported to have spasmolytic properties (Hall and Clarke, 1983).

Anticholinergic drugs, such as atropine or glycopyrrolate, reduce gastric secretions and decrease gastric motility (Adams, 1982). Because of these properties it has been suggested that they will reduce the incidence and severity of the acid aspiration syndrome (Mendelson, 1946; Marx, 1973; Short, 1987). Unfortunately, these agents also decrease tone in the gastro-oesophageal sphincter, while pyloric sphincter tone is increased (Strombeck and Harrold, 1985). This will have the effect of delaying gastric emptying and may increase the risk of gastric reflux (Gibbs and Modell, 1986).

Metoclopramide, a drug which blocks dopamine receptors and facilitates cholinergic transmission, may be more effective than anticholinergic agents in preventing gastric aspiration. This drug has anti-emetic properties, promotes gastric emptying and increases the barrier pressure across the lower oesophageal sphincter (Flacke and Flacke, 1986; Trim, 1987).

Induction

Intravenous administration of a rapidly acting barbiturate is relatively safe in patients with minimal circulatory impairment. This method of induction permits rapid control of the airway and will reduce the risk of aspiration in patients liable to vomit or regurgitate during the induction process. When peripheral circulatory failure is present, neuroleptanalgesic combinations may be safer than barbiturates for induction as they cause less cardiovascular depression. Inhalational induction techniques are preferable in critically ill patients because they allow precise and reliable control of the level of anaesthesia without causing acute changes in the physiological status of the patient. A disadvantage of inhalational induction is the increased risk of vomition and subsequent aspiration. The choice of inhalational anaesthetic is not as important as the method of deployment. One desirable characteristic of an inhalational agent for use in patients with gastrointestinal disturbance is the ability to cause rapid loss of consciousness with little or no associated cardiopulmonary depression. In this respect, isoflurane may be the most suitable agent.

Following induction of anaesthesia, the patient should be intubated as rapidly as possible using a cuffed endotracheal tube. When regurgitation is likely to occur during induction, the patient should be supported in sternal recumbency with the head and neck elevated throughout the procedure. Sellick's manoeuvre, which involves applying pressure to the cricoid cartilage to occlude the oesophagus during induction, may be used to advantage in this situation (Sellick, 1961). If regurgitation or vomition occurs, the head should be lowered to facilitate drainage of material from the buccal cavity and pharynx. Suctioning and swabbing will assist in débridement of these areas.

Maintenance

Anaesthesia can be maintained safely using a volatile anaesthetic such as halothane or isoflurane delivered in oxygen. Isoflurane has advantages over halothane when cardiac dysrhythmias are present because it does not sensitize the myocardium to catecholamines (Eger, 1984). For low risk patients, no major modifications in technique are required. For seriously ill patients, the lowest possible concentration of the volatile anaesthetic agent should be used to minimize cardiopulmonary depression. The concentration of the volatile agent can be reduced by the simultaneous administration of nitrous oxide (DeYoung and Sawyer, 1980). Nitrous oxide should be avoided if any closed, gas-filled pockets exist or if arterial oxygenation is marginal (Booth, 1982).

Positive pressure ventilation helps to maintain adequate alveolar ventilation in extremely debilitated patients or when diaphragmatic excursions are hampered by increased abdominal pressure. The safe use of positive pressure ventilation requires familiarity with its potential adverse effects and methods by which these effects may be minimized (Hall and Clarke, 1983).

Balanced anaesthetic techniques provide the ultimate in safe anaesthetic management of critically ill patients. These techniques require considerable experience to master and are potentially unsafe in the hands of an untrained individual. Recently, balanced techniques involving intravenous infusions of either opioid agents or ketamine have been advocated in severely debilitated dogs (Yamane *et al.*, 1985; Benson *et al.*, 1987).

All vital signs should be monitored at 5-minute intervals or less. Continuous monitoring of the patient is recommended when parameters are changing rapidly. Measurement of arterial and central venous pressure is useful when circulatory disorders necessitate extensive fluid replacement therapy. Periodic assessment of the haematocrit and total serum solids will also provide some indication of the effectiveness of fluid therapy and facilitate rational adjustments in estimated requirements. Serial arterial blood gas analysis will permit correction of the metabolic status of the patient as well as indicating the ventilatory status.

Recovery

In patients that are likely to vomit or regurgitate during recovery, the endotracheal tube should be maintained in place with the cuff inflated for as long as it will be tolerated. If regurgitation occurs, the oropharynx should be thoroughly débrided with absorbent swabs or by the use of surgical suction. The endotracheal tube should be removed with the cuff still inflated once the animal is swallowing vigorously.

Close monitoring should continue throughout the recovery period and supplementary oxygen, fluids and analgesic drugs should be administered as necessary. One extremely serious potential complication of surgery is septic shock. Although septic shock may be associated with many different forms of infection, it occurs most commonly after major gastrointestinal surgery (Ledingham and McArdle, 1978). Monitoring should be performed with this in mind and patients should be treated early if signs of sepsis become apparent.

REFERENCES

Adams, H. R. (1982). In *Veterinary Pharmacology and Therapeutics*, p. 127. Ames: Iowa State University Press.

Ali, H. H. (1985). *Clinics in Anesthesiology* 3, 447.

Baden, J. M., Serra, M., Fuginaga, M. and Mazze, R. I. (1987). *Anesthesiology* 61, 660.

Bastron, R. D. (1986). In *37th Refresher Course Lectures of the ASA (Oct.)* 243, 1.

Bastron, R. D. and Deutsch, S. (1976). In *Anesthesia and the Kidney*, p. 29. New York: Grune and Stratton.

Benson, G. J. and Brock, K. A. (1980). *Journal of Veterinary Pharmacology and Therapeutics* 3, 187.

Benson, G. J. and Thurmon, J. C. (1987). In *Principles and Practice of Veterinary Anesthesia*, p. 237. Baltimore: Williams and Wilkins.

Benson, G. J., Thurmon, J. C., Tranquilli, W. J. and Corbin, J. E. (1987). *American Journal of Veterinary Research* 48, 1372.

Berry, A. J. (1981). *Anesthesiology* 55, 655.

Bidwai, A. V., Stanley, T. H., Bloomer, H. A. and Blatnick, R. A. (1975). *Anesthesia and Analgesia* 54, 357.

Biewenga, W. J., deVries, H. W., Stockhof, A. A. and deBruyne, J. J. (1978). *Veterinary Anesthesia* 5, 8.

Bone, R. C., Fisher, C. J., Clemmer, T. P., Slotman, G. J., Metz, C. A., Balk, R. A. and the Methyl-prednisolone Severe Sepsis Study Group. (1987). *New England Journal of Medicine* 317, 653.

Booth, N. H. (1982). In *Veterinary Pharmacology and Therapeutics*, 5th edn, p. 241. Ames, Iowa: Iowa State University Press.

Branch, R. A., Morgan, M. H., James, J. and Read, A. E. (1976). *Gut* 17, 975.

Brown, B. R. (1972). *Anesthesiology* 36, 458.

Burrows, C. F. and Bovee, K. C. (1978). *Journal of the American Veterinary Medical Association* 172, 801.

Card, B., McCulloch, R. J. and Pratt, D. A. H. (1972). *Postgraduate Medical Journal* **48**, 123.

Carter, S. W. and Mercer, A. E. (1987). *Proceedings of the American College of Veterinary Anesthesiologists*, p. 2. Atlanta, Georgia.

Chapman, R. L., Modell, J. H., Ruiz, B. C., Calderwood, H. W., Hood, C. I. and Graves, S. A. (1974). *Anesthesia and Analgesia* **53**, 556.

Child, K. J., Davis, B., Dodds, M. G. and Twissell, D. J. (1972a). *British Journal of Pharmacology* **46**, 189.

Child, K. J., Gibson, W., Hornby, G. and Hart, J. W. (1972b) *Postgraduate Medical Journal* **48**, 37.

Clark, A. M. (1980). *Veterinary Record* **106**, 146.

Court, M. H., Dodman, N. H. and Seeler, D. C. (1985). *Veterinary Clinics of North America* **15**, 1041.

Cousins, M. K. (1984). In *35th Refresher Course Lectures of the ASA (Oct.)* New Orleans, Louisiana **204**, 1.

Cuschieri, A. (1980). In *General Anaesthesia*, 4th edn, vol. 2, p. 1697. London: Butterworths.

Davis, B. and Pearce, D. R. (1972). *Postgraduate Medical Journal* **48**, 13.

Deutsch, S. (1973). *Veterinary Clinics of North America* **3**, 57.

DeYoung, D. J. and Sawyer, D. C. (1980). *Journal of the American Animal Hospital Association* **16**, 1265.

Dibartola, S. P. (1980). *Compendium of Continuing Education* **11**, 952.

Dixon, S. H., Nolan, S. P., Stewart, S. and Morrow, A. G. (1970). *Anesthesia and Analgesia* **49**, 331.

Dodman, N. H., Engelking, L. R. and Anwer, M. S. (1987). In *Principles and Practice of Veterinary Anesthesia*, p. 221. Baltimore: Williams and Wilkins.

Dodman, N. H., Seeler, D. C. and Court, M. H. (1984). *British Veterinary Journal* **140**, 505.

Dodman, N. H., Seeler, D. C., Norman, W. and Court, M. H. (1987). *British Veterinary Journal* **143**, 291.

Don, H. F., Dieppa, R. A. and Taylor, P. (1975). *Anesthesiology* **42**, 745.

Dundee, J. W. and McCaughey, W. (1980). In *General Anaesthesia*, 4th edn, vol. 2, p. 923. London: Butterworths.

Duvaldstein, P., Lebrault, C., Terestchenko, M. C. and Strumza, P. (1983). In *Clinical Experiences with Norcuron*, p. 180. Amsterdam: Excerpta Medica.

Eger, E. I. (1981). *Isoflurane (Forane): a Compendium and Reference*. Madison, Wisconsin: Airco Inc.

Eger, E. I. (1984). In *Isoflurane (Forane): a Compendium and Reference*. Madison, Wisconsin: Anaquest.

Erhardt, W., Stephan, M., Schatzmann, U., Westermayr, R.,

Schindele, M., Murisier, N and Blumel, G. (1986). *Journal of the Association of Veterinary Anaesthetists* **14**, 90.

Fewell, J. and Bond, G. C. (1980). *Anesthesiology* **52**, 408.

Flacke, W. E. and Flacke, J. W. (1986). In *Drug Interactions in Anesthesia*, 2nd edn, p, 173. Philadelphia: Lea and Febiger.

Ghoneim, M. M. and Pandya, H. (1975). *Anesthesiology* **42**, 545.

Gibbs, C. P. and Modell, J. H. (1986). In *Anesthesia*, 2nd edn, p. 2039. New York: Churchill Livingstone.

Gorman, H. M. and Craythorne, N. W. B. (1966). *Acta Anaesthesiologica Scandinavica (Supplement)* **24**, 11.

Grauer, G. F. (1985). *Compendium on Continuing Education* **7**, 32.

Groeger, J. S., Carlon, G. C. and Howland, W. S. (1983). *Critical Care Medicine* **2**, 650.

Hall, L. W. & Clarke, K. W. (1983). In *Veterinary Anaesthesia*, 8th edn, pp. 51, 74, 141, 305. London: Baillière Tindall.

Hardie, E. M. and Rawlings, C. A. (1983). *Compendium on Continuing Education* **5**, 483.

Hardie, E. M., Rawlings, C. A. and Collins, L. G. (1985). *Journal of the American Animal Hospital Association* **21**, 691.

Hart, R. (1971). In *Proceedings of the Association of Veterinary Anaesthetists of Great Britain and Ireland* **2**, 14.

Haskins, S. C., Farver, T. B. and Patz, J. D. (1985). *American Journal of Veterinary Research* **46**, 1855.

Haskins, S. C., Farver, T. B. and Patz, J. D. (1986). *American Journal of Veterinary Research* **47**, 795.

Haskins, S. C., Patz, J. D. and Farver, T. B. (1986). *American Journal of Veterinary Research* **47**, 636.

Haskins, S.C., Patz, J. D., Copland, S. Y., Yamamoto, Y. & Orima, H. (1987). *Proceedings of the American College of Veterinary Anesthesiologists*, p. 1. Atlanta, Georgia.

Hinshaw, L., Peduzzi, P., Young, E., Sprung, C., Shatney, C., Sheagren, J., Wilson, M. and Haakenson, C. (1987). *New England Journal of Medicine* **317**, 659.

Hursh, D., Gelman, S. and Bradley, E. L. (1987). *Anesthesiology* **67**, 701.

Ilkiw, J. E., Sampson, D. and Cutler, D. (1985). *Proceedings of the 2nd International Congress of Veterinary Anesthesia*, p. 118. Sacramento, California.

Jones, A. E., Schafter, D. F., Ferenci, P. and Pappas, S. C. (1985). *Hepatology* **4**, 1235.

Jones, D. J., Stehling, L. C. and Zauder, H. L. (1979). *Anesthesiology* **51**, 430.

Kelman, J. W. (1969). *Surgery* **66**, 886.

Klein, L. V. (1987). In *Principles and Practice of Veterinary Anesthesia*, p. 143. Baltimore, Maryland: Williams & Wilkins.

Klide, A. M., Calderwood, H. W. and Soma, L. R. (1975). *American Journal of Veterinary Research* **36**, 931.

Knight, A. P. (1980). *Journal of the American Veterinary Medical Association* **176**, 454.

Kolata, R. J. and Rawlings, C. A. (1982). *Journal of the American Animal Hospital Association* **43**, 2196.

Lebrault, C., Berger, J. L., D'Hollander, A. A., Gomeni, R., Henzel, D. and Duvaldstein, P. (1985). *Anesthesiology* **62**, 601.

Ledingham, I. McA. and McArdle, C. S. (1978). *Lancet* **ii**, 470.

Ledingham, I. McA. and Routh, G. S. (1979). *British Journal of Hospital Medicine* **22**, 472.

Lewis, A. A. G. (1963). In *Clinical Physiology*, 2nd edn, p. 160. Oxford: Blackwell.

Lumb, W. V. and Jones, E. W. (1984). In *Veterinary Anesthesia*, 2nd edn. pp. 165, 279, 567. Philadelphia: Lea & Febiger.

Lunding, M. (1965). *Acta Anaesthesiologica Scandinavia (Supplement)* **15**, 139.

Marx, G. F. (1973). In *Clinical Anesthesia*, No. 2. Philadelphia: F. A. Davis Co.

Mazze, R. I. (1984). *Canadian Anaesthetists Society Journal* **31**, S16.

McDonell, W. N. and Van Gorder, J. (1982). In *Proceedings of the American College of Veterinary Anesthesiologists*, p. 28. Las Vegas, Nevada.

Mendelson, C. L. (1946). *American Journal of Obstetrics and Gynecology* **52**, 181.

Miller, R. D. (1983). In *34th Refresher Course Lectures of the ASA (Oct)*. Atlanta. Georgia **220**, 1.

Muir, W. W. (1982). *Journal of the American Veterinary Medical Association* **180**, 729.

Orton, E. C. and Muir, W. W. (1983). *American Journal of Veterinary Research* **44**, 1512.

Osborne, C. A. and Polzin, D. J. (1983a). *Compendium on Continuing Education* **5**, 497.

Osborne, C. A. and Polzin, D. J. (1983b). *Compendium on Continuing Education* **5**, 561.

Pascoe, P. J. (1987). In *Principles and Practice of Veterinary Anesthesia*, ed. C. E. Short, p. 558. Baltimore: Williams and Wilkins.

Pedersoli, W. M. (1977). *Journal of the American Animal Hospital Association* **13**, 242.

Peters, W. P., Friedman, P. A., Johnson, M. W. and Mitch, W. E. (1981). *Lancet* **i**, 529.

Polzin, D. J. and Osborne, C. A. (1985). In *Handbook of Small Animal Therapeutics*, p. 333. New York: Churchill Livingstone.

Priano, L. L. (1984). In *35th Refresher Course Lectures of the ASA (Oct)*. New Orleans, Louisiana **240**, 1.

Pugh, D. M. (1964). *Veterinary Record* **76**, 439.
Raffe, M. R. (1987). In *Principles and Practice of Veterinary Anesthesia*, p. 480. Baltimore: Williams & Wilkins.
Read, A. E. (1979). *British Journal of Hospital Medicine* **22**, 490.
Sams, R. A. and Muir, W. W. (1986). *Proceedings of the Veterinary Midwest Anesthesia Conference*. Urbana, Illinois.
Sawyer, D. C. (1982). In *The Practice of Small Animal Anesthesia*, pp. 1, 8, 13. Philadelphia: Saunders.
Sear, J. W. (1984). In *Pharmacokinetics of Anaesthesia*, p. 64. Boston: Blackwell.
Seeler, D. C. and Thurmon, J. C. (1985). In *Handbook of Small Animal Therapeutics*, p. 21. New York: Churchill Livingstone.
Seeler, D. C., Dodman, N. H., Norman, W. M. and Court, M. H. (1987). *British Veterinary Journal* **143**, 97.
Sellick, B. A. (1961). *Lancet* **ii**, 404.
Shoemaker, W. C. and Hauser, C. J. (1979). *Critical Care Medicine* **7**, 117.
Short, C. E. (1987). In *Principles and Practice of Veterinary Anesthesia*, ed. C. E. Short, p. 18. Baltimore: Williams and Wilkins.
Sladen, R. (1982). In *33rd Refresher Course Lectures of the ASA (Oct.)* Las Vegas, Nevada **211**, 1.
Sollmann, T. (1948). In *A Manual of Pharmacology*, 7th edn, p. 228. London: Saunders.
Spence, A. A. (1980). In *General Anaesthesia*, 4th edn, vol. 1, p. 591. London: Butterworths
Sprung, C. L. Caralis, P. V., Marcial, E. H., Pierce, M., Gelbard, M. A., Long, W. M., Duncan, R. C., Tendler, M. D. and Karpf, M. (1984). *New England Journal of Medicine* **311**, 1137.
Stephenson, J. C., Blevins, D. I. and Christie, G. J. (1978). *Veterinary Medicine Small Animal Clinician* **3**, 303.
Strombeck, D. R. and Harrold, D. (1985). *American Journal of Veterinary Research* **46**, 965.
Strunin, L. (1980). In *General Anaesthesia*, 4th edn, vol. 1, p. 779. London: Butterworths.
Trim, C. M. (1979). *Compendium on Continuing Education* **1**, 11, 843.
Trim, C. M. (1987). In *Principles and Practice of Veterinary Anesthesia*, ed. C. E. Short, p. 261. Baltimore: Williams and Wilkins.
Tyler, R. D., Qualls, C. W., Heald, R. D., Cowell, R. L. and Clinkenbeard, K. D. (1987). *Journal of the American Veterinary Medical Association* **191**, 1095.
Waxman, K., Shoemaker, W. C. and Lippmann, M. (1980). *Anesthesia and Analgesia* **59**, 355.
White, P. F. (1984). *35th Refresher Course Lectures of the ASA*. Chicago, Illinois **505**, 1.
Yamane, Y., Matsuda, D., Nakaniwa, S., Sato, N., Haruna, A.,

Shibazaki, F., Yamagata, H. and Noishiki, Y. (1985). In *Proceedings of the 2nd International Congress of Veterinary Anesthesia*, p. 128. Sacramento, California.

Zarowitz, H. and Friedman, I. S. (1957). *New England Journal of Medicine* **57**, 1922.

Zimmerman, H. J. (1978). In *Hepatotoxicity*, p. 546. New York: Appleton-Century-Crofts.

9

Anaesthesia for patients with endocrine disease

Endocrine disease is frequently encountered in small animal patients requiring general anaesthesia for either medical or surgical purposes. Most often, the procedure is unrelated to the primary endocrine disturbance; however, a number of endocrinopathies require specific surgical treatment. These may include patients with hyperthyroidism, phaeochromocytoma, pancreatic insulin-secreting tumour and cortisol-secreting tumour of the adrenal cortex (Peterson, Birchhard and Mehlhaff, 1984).

More than one endocrine disturbance may occur in the same patient and these disturbances are often inter-related. For instance, hyperadrenocorticism often occurs in association with diabetes mellitus in man and dog (Peterson, Nesbitt and Schaer, 1981). Other non-endocrine diseases may also occur in association with the primary endocrine disorder and affect the animal's medical management. Pancreatitis is often diagnosed in diabetic patients, requiring specific medical therapy, while stress-inducing events, such as systemic infections, pregnancy or surgery, will increase the insulin requirements of diabetics (Nelson and Feldman, 1986).

Most endocrine disorders adversely affect the homeostatic control mechanisms of the body. General anaesthesia and surgery may further compromise homeostasis or even worsen the primary endocrine disturbance. An understanding of the pathophysiological changes associated with endocrine disease and of the inter-relationships between endocrine disease and non-endocrine influences is essential to the successful medical, surgical and anaesthetic management of these cases. This chapter will focus on the preanaesthetic assessment, preparation and anaesthetic management of small animal patients with endocrine disease.

161

PANCREAS

Diabetes mellitus

Diabetes mellitus is probably the most common endocrinopathy in the dog, while a mild form of this disease is occasionally diagnosed in the cat (Fraser and Mays, 1986). Diabetes is a chronic disorder of carbohydrate metabolism resulting from relative or absolute insulin deficiency (Nelson and Feldman, 1986). The commonest form of canine diabetes resembles human type I, insulin-dependent diabetes, while the majority of cats may have non-insulin-dependent diabetes (human type II). Canine diabetes can occur at any age in either sex, but is most common in middle-aged to older females (Nelson and Feldman, 1986). Feline diabetes is also more common in older individuals but occurs most frequently in males (Feldman and Nelson, 1986). Hormonally induced diabetes mellitus is well documented in dogs and cats, and may result from increased plasma concentrations of any of the diabetogenic hormones, including glucocorticoids, adrenaline, glucagon or growth hormone (Nelson and Feldman, 1986). Increased progesterone levels in pregnant animals or exogenous administration of progestins may also antagonize insulin by stimulation of growth hormone secretion (Eigenman, 1981).

Hypoinsulinaemia and peripheral tissue insensitivity to insulin result in decreased peripheral tissue carbohydrate, amino acid and triglyceride utilization. A fasting hyperglycaemia is one of the more consistent clinical findings. Other abnormalities related to this condition include polydipsia, polyuria, polyphagia and weight loss. Commonly, subclinical (or latent) diabetes may be exacerbated by concurrent disease, including pancreatitis, congestive heart failure or urinary tract infections, or by oestrus and certain medications (Nelson and Feldman, 1986). Chronic hyperglycaemia may result in a number of secondary complications, the most common in the dog being cataract formation.

Insulin-dependent diabetes mellitus is normally controlled by the administration of exogenous insulin, usually of the intermediate-acting (isophane insulin (NPH) or zinc insulin (lente)) or long-acting (protamine zinc insulin (PZI)) form. Blood glucose control regimens using multiple daily injections of intermediate-acting insulins are commonly advocated to maintain a euglycaemic state in the dog (Nelson and Feldman, 1986).

There is much evidence linking chronic hyperglycaemia and the end-stage organ pathology responsible for the long-term complications of diabetes mellitus in humans (Winegrad, 1986). Such pathological changes are considered to be responsible for the majority of perioperative problems in human diabetics (Ammon,

1987). These changes include coronary artery disease, hypertension, cardiac autonomic neuropathy, impaired ventricular function, unexpected sudden death, intrinsic diabetic renal disease, urosepsis, delayed gastric emptying, stiff joint syndrome and abnormal counter-regulatory response to hypoglycaemia (Ammon, 1987). The majority of these pathological changes are either unreported or poorly documented in small animals. This may be associated with the relatively short duration of the disease process in most small animal diabetics. It remains to be seen whether these complications develop in veterinary patients with chronic diabetes mellitus (>5 years), particularly in those patients with poor blood glucose control.

A number of conditions commonly associated with diabetes have been reported to complicate the anaesthetic management of small animal patients, including hepatopathy, prerenal uraemia, urinary tract infection and ketoacidosis (Brock, 1983).

Preanaesthetic assessment and preparation. Diabetic small animals should be admitted to the hospital at least 24 hours prior to elective surgery to allow assessment of the patient's metabolic status. Unstabilized diabetics may present with metabolic derangements ranging from mild hyperglycaemia, dehydration and hypokalaemia to severe hyperglycaemia and ketoacidosis or hyperosmolar coma. In addition, diabetics apparently stabilized on insulin may occasionally present with hypoglycaemia. Clinical pathology data, including fasting blood glucose, ketones, serum electrolytes, blood urea nitrogen, creatinine and acid-base balance should be evaluated in these patients on admission. Abnormalities should be corrected using appropriate intravenous fluid therapy and supplemental administration of regular insulin as required.

Animals that are severely hyperglycaemic (blood glucose >300 mg dl^{-1}) or are ketoacidotic should be stabilized by intramuscular injections of regular insulin at 0.1 units kg^{-1} every hour until blood glucose is within the normal range (70–110 mg dl^{-1}) and continued at 0.5 units/kg every 6–8 hours as needed (Chastain, 1981). Subcutaneous administration of insulin is not recommended in animals with circulatory compromise or during the perioperative period because of variations in skin blood flow and erratic absorption. Absorption from subcutaneous sites may be increased by application of heat or shivering and is retarded by hypothermia or sympathetic-induced vasoconstriction.

As an alternative to low dose intramuscular insulin therapy, animals that require more immediate stabilization, such as prior to emergency surgery, may be administered regular insulin by constant intravenous infusion. Ideally this should be done using a calibrated intravenous infusion pump, although a paediatric infusion set with a volumetric reservoir chamber will suffice. Ten to 15 units of regular insulin is usually added to 1 litre of infusate (normally 0.9% saline or 5% dextrose in water) and insulin infusion initiated at a rate of 0.05–0.1 units kg^{-1} h^{-1}. The administration rate is then adjusted to maintain euglycaemia (Chastain, 1981).

It should be remembered that up to 50% of the insulin added to the infusate will bind to the walls of the plastic or glass container and administration set (Petty and Cunningham, 1974). Variations in the administration rate of insulin to the patient with each container of fluids may result. This effect should be minimized by initially running 50 ml of solution through the i.v. set to stabilize the insulin concentration. The use of a separate insulin infusion container and administration set as opposed to periodically adding insulin to the animal's regular intravenous fluids is also recommended. Absorption of insulin to the fluid container may be reduced by adding plasma or a gelatin-based plasma expander to the insulin solution (Kraegen *et al.*, 1975). The addition of 10 ml of the patient's blood to 1 litre of infusate has also been recommended for this purpose (Brock, 1983).

Diabetic animals are prone to infections (Nelson and Feldman, 1986). A complete blood count should be taken preoperatively to detect subclinical sepsis which, if found, should be treated with appropriate antibiotic therapy. Scrupulous aseptic technique should also be used during any invasive procedure including intravenous catheterization.

A complete biochemical profile is a useful preoperative screening process for diabetic small animals to detect concurrent major organ disease, especially those diseases involving the liver and kidneys. Cirrhosis or hepatomegaly resulting from fatty infiltration of the liver is common in diabetics. Urosepsis and prerenal azotaemia are also frequently diagnosed. The extent of functional organ impairment should be assessed preoperatively.

Food should be withheld from diabetic patents for 12 hours prior to induction to reduce the incidence of vomition and aspiration. Unfortunately, since insulin administration in the insulin-dependent diabetic is normally followed by food intake, the animal's normal morning insulin regimen must be altered or intravenous glucose administered to prevent hypoglycaemia. Such regimens will be discussed in the next section.

Anaesthetic management. The principles of management of diabetic patients during anaesthesia include:

1. The prevention of hypoglycaemia.
2. The prevention of ketoacidosis.

3. Control of severe hyperglycaemia.
4. Maintenance of normal fluid and electrolyte balance.

Although commonly used anaesthetic agents may affect glucose metabolism, their direct effect on blood glucose homeostasis is modest in comparison to the stress response associated with anaesthesia and surgery (Clarke, 1970; Hardie, Rawlings and George, 1985). In general, anaesthesia and surgery have been shown to increase adrenaline, noradrenaline, cortisol, growth hormone and glucagon levels. Insulin levels are usually unaffected but a decrease in peripheral insulin effectiveness is common (Bevan, 1980). Anaesthetic agents which minimize these effects are preferred and include the commonly used sedative drugs (such as acepromazine), the barbiturates, the methylethyl ether inhalation agents (methoxyflurane, enflurane and isoflurane) and nitrous oxide. Agents which are markedly hyperglycaemic, such as xylazine ketamine, ether and cyclopropane, should be avoided (Bevan, 1980; Booth, 1982; Hsu and Hembrough, 1982). Administration of glucocorticoids should be avoided because of their anti-insulin effects. These agents may compound immunosuppression which is a common feature of diabetes mellitus.

Many different regimens have been advocated for control of blood glucose in diabetic surgical patients. These methods vary in the degree to which blood glucose is allowed to vary from normal, ranging from so-called 'tight' control regimens in which glucose and insulin are infused continuously during surgery; to 'non-tight' control regimens in which no food, glucose or insulin is given on the day of surgery. Unfortunately, while 'tight' control regimens are probably ideal for the unstable, ketoacidotic patient, these methods can be fraught with complications and are labour intensive, particularly if an intravenous infusion pump is unavailable. Likewise, 'non-tight' control regimens may be satisfactory in patients that are only insulin depleted but may be suboptimal in insulin-deficient diabetics. These latter patients may become progressively hyperglycaemic and ketotic in the face of insulin withdrawal.

Peterson *et al.* (1984) have suggested a blood glucose control regimen which is a compromise between simplicity and complexity, and appears to be both convenient and effective for the majority of stable insulin-dependent diabetics. With this regimen, the animal is given insulin and fed as usual on the day before surgery. Food is withheld from midnight that day, and surgery scheduled for early morning the next day to allow for intensive postoperative management. Approximately 1 hour before surgery, a blood glucose is taken, one-half of the usual morning dose of insulin is administered, and the animal is started on an intravenous infusion of 5% dextrose in water. If the blood glucose is greater than 300 mg dl^{-1}, then a supplemental dose of regular insulin (0.25–0.5 units kg^{-1} i.m.) is administered.

During surgery, the blood glucose is monitored at regular intervals, preferably hourly. This is most rapidly and conveniently accomplished using glucose oxidase test strips. This assay provides semiquantitative determinations of blood glucose concentration within 2 minutes using a small drop of venous blood. Inexpensive but accurate electronic blood glucose monitoring devices are also available (Brock, 1983). If the blood glucose concentration is greater than 300 mg dl^{-1}, then additional regular insulin (0.25–0.5 units kg i.m.) should be administered. Rarely, patients become hypoglycaemic. However, if the blood glucose decreases to less than 100 mg dl^{-1}, the rate of dextrose infusion should be increased.

Unstabilized diabetics should be maintained during and following surgery with a 'tight' blood glucose control regimen using an intravenous infusion of dextrose and regular insulin as previously described. Blood glucose determinations should be more frequent than for stabilized diabetics. Periodic intraoperative blood gas analysis is also advised, particularly if the animal was ketoacidotic preoperatively. A balanced electrolyte solution should be administered in addition to the dextrose–insulin infusion in order to maintain the fluid and electrolyte requirements of the animal.

Postoperative management of the diabetic patient depends on the time that oral intake is resumed. Administration of dextrose should be continued with regular insulin given intramuscularly every 6 hours to maintain blood glucose between 150–250 mg dl^{-1}. Unstable diabetics should be monitored intensively like other critically ill patients with particular attention given to acid–base status and fluid electrolyte balance. In most cases, oral feeding and a routine insulin administration schedule can be resumed on the first or second day after surgery.

Pancreatic insulin-secreting tumour (insulinoma)

Insulin-secreting tumour of the pancreas (or insulinoma) is a well-recognized endocrine neoplasm in the dog resulting in clinical signs related to hypoglycaemia. Insulinomas are most often diagnosed in middle-aged to older dogs (Leifer, 1986). The majority of these tumours are malignant with about 45% of dogs having detectable metastasis at the time of surgery (Peterson *et al.*, 1984).

Clinical signs are related to the degree and duration of hypoglycaemia. Affected dogs may demonstrate grand mal seizures, posterior paresis, collapse, shaking, trembling, generalized weakness, ataxia, focal facial seizures, polyphagia, polyuria, polydipsia, behavioural changes or status epilepticus. Multiple signs are common and become more frequent as the disease progresses (Leifer, 1986).

Diagnosis of insulin-secreting tumour is based on demonstrating a relationship between clinical signs and hypoglycaemia, and the detection of an absolute or relative hyperinsulinaemia. Evaluation of the insulin : glucose ratio and the amended insulin : glucose ratio is helpful in cases of relative hyperinsulinaemia (Leifer, 1986). Other causes of hypoglycaemia should be ruled out.

Surgical removal of the primary tumour, and if possible, resection of any metastatic disease is the treatment of choice in these patients (Mehlhaff *et al.*, 1985). Medical methods of controlling hypoglycaemia have been used if the owner declines surgical intervention, for temporary control of blood glucose preoperatively or if hypoglycaemia recurs postoperatively (Leifer, Peterson and Matus, 1986). These methods include frequent feeding with complex carbohydrates alone or in combination with oral diazoxide therapy. This drug is thought to inhibit pancreatic insulin secretion directly, enhance adrenaline-induced glycogenolysis, and inhibit glucose uptake by the tissues. The most common adverse effects of diazoxide therapy are vomition and anorexia (Leifer, 1986).

Preanaesthetic assessment and preparation. It is important to avoid further episodes of clinical hypoglycaemia before surgery. Fasting blood glucose levels should be routinely assessed and, if indicated (blood glucose < 70 mg dl^{-1}), medical management should be instituted by frequent feeding with or without diazoxide. Preoperative administration of diazoxide is useful for a number of reasons. First, a positive response to this drug helps substantiate the diagnosis of insulin-secreting tumour (Higgins, 1979). Second, animals which respond to this drug need not be euthanatized if a non-resectable tumour is found during surgery. Medical therapy may be effective for controlling hypoglycaemia in these patients for variable periods (Peterson *et al.*, 1984).

Occasionally, hypoglycaemia persists despite conservative medical therapy. Preoperative fasting of these patients may also be associated with unacceptably low blood glucose concentrations. In these cases, the patient should be started on an intravenous infusion of 5% dextrose in water. The concentration of dextrose in the infusate may need to be increased in steps of 5% until the blood glucose level is greater than 60 mg dl^{-1} (Muir *et al.*, 1983). Bolus doses of glucose should be avoided because of the possibility of stimulating excessive insulin release and causing severe, paroxysmal hypoglycaemia.

Preoperative administration of glucocorticoids may also be useful in patients with persistent hypoglycaemia since these agents increase hepatic gluconeogenesis and inhibit tissue glucose uptake

(Leifer and Peterson, 1984). Large doses of glucocorticoids should be avoided before surgery because they delay wound healing and increase the risks of infection.

All dogs should be fasted from midnight on the day before surgery. A 5–20% dextrose infusion should be started at this time. The administration rate should meet the maintenance fluid requirements of the animal (normally 80 ml kg^{-1} daily), while the concentration of dextrose solution should be adjusted to maintain euglycaemia.

Anaesthetic management. The maintenance of euglycaemia in the anaesthetized patient with insulin-secreting tumour is of paramount importance because of the serious adverse consequences of hypoglycaemia. A prolonged period of neuroglucopenia can result in irreversible damage to glucose-dependent neural tissue, particularly the cerebral cortex, basal ganglia, and rostral medulla. Peripheral neuropathy has also been documented in dogs (Leifer, 1986). The development of these changes is undetectable in anaesthetized patients.

A rational approach to the selection of anaesthetic agents for use in patients with insulinoma would be to choose agents that decrease cerebral glucose utilization (Suffecol, 1980). These agents would tend to have a protective effect on neural tissue during hypoglycaemic episodes. In this regard, the thiobarbiturates and the volatile inhalational agents may be the agents of choice for induction and maintenance of anaesthesia because they appear to decrease cerebral glucose metabolism (Suffecol, 1980). Halothane and enflurane may also be beneficial because these agents have been shown to decrease glucose-stimulated insulin release (Gingevich, Wright and Paradise, 1980; Ewart, Rusy and Bradford, 1981). High concentrations of enflurane (> 3%), ketamine, tiletamine, and analeptic agents such as doxapram will increase cerebral metabolic rate and therefore should be avoided.

As mentioned previously, it is of the utmost importance to be able to recognize and treat hypoglycaemia in the anaesthetized insulinoma patient before development of irreversible central nervous system damage. A rapid fall in blood glucose concentration in the awake patient will stimulate hypothalamic glucoreceptors and cause an increase in adrenergic activity (Leifer, 1986). This effect, although obtunded during anaesthesia, may become evident as a paroxysmal increase in heart rate and arterial pressure unrelated to the depth of anaesthesia or surgical manipulation.

The safest means to avoid intraoperative hypoglycaemia is to routinely administer 5–20% dextrose intravenously throughout the procedure and measure the blood glucose concentration every

30 minutes using one of the rapid assay techniques previously described (Peterson *et al.*, 1984). The concentration and rate of administration of the dextrose solution should be adjusted to maintain the blood glucose concentration above 70 mg dl^{-1}. Additional fluid requirements may be met by administering a balanced electrolyte solution, such as lactated Ringer's solution, in conjunction with the dextrose infusion.

Recently, a feedback-controlled dextrose/insulin infusion device, called an artificial pancreas, has become commercially available for the intraoperative management of human patients with insulinoma. This device continuously monitors plasma glucose concentrations and can administer either dextrose or insulin to maintain plasma glucose in a predetermined range (Muir *et al.*, 1983). This device has the disadvantages of being expensive, large, complex and of requiring an experienced operator (Pulver *et al.*, 1980).

Some authors contend that dextrose should not be administered during surgery unless the patient becomes hypoglycaemic because this will mask 'hyperglycaemic rebound' a sudden increase in blood glucose concentration which may indicate successful removal of the tumour (van Heerden, Edis and Service, 1979; Suffecol, 1980). Unfortunately this technique requires frequent monitoring of blood glucose levels (at least every 15 minues) to avoid sudden episodes of hypoglycaemia which are often associated with physical manipulation of the tumour. Using this technique, nine out of 35 human patients undergoing insulinoma resection developed severe hypoglycaemia requiring dextrose infusion. (Muir *et al.*, 1983). In addition, the study by Muir *et al.* (1983) determined that 'hyperglycaemic rebound' was not helpful in determining the adequacy of surgical excision.

When the tumour is removed, the dextrose infusion should be terminated if the patient becomes hyperglycaemic. A temporary functional diabetes mellitus associated with transient suppression of residual beta-cell activity is common in patients following successful removal of the insulin-producing tumour (Peterson *et al.*, 1984). Blood glucose concentrations should be monitored frequently (every 60 minutes) for at least 24 hours after surgery since the return of hypoglycaemia may indicate functional metastatic tissue. Persistent hyperglycaemia or the onset of ketonaemia should be treated with supplemental insulin administration.

Pancreatitis is a common sequela to pancreatic surgery. Because of this it has been suggesed that food and water should be withheld for 48–72 hours following surgery (Peterson *et al.*, 1984). Fluid balance should be maintained with intravenous fluids during this time. Serum amylase and lipase activity should be determined on a daily basis to ensure a return to normal levels.

ADRENAL CORTEX

Hypoadrenocorticism (adrenocortical insufficiency)

Hypoadrenocorticism or adrenocortical insufficiency results from insufficient production of glucocorticoid, mineralocorticoid, or both. Spontaneous hypoadrenocorticism is a relatively uncommon endocrinopathy in dogs, most often diagnosed in young to middle-aged females. It is extremely rare in the cat (Schrader, 1986).

Primary adrenocortical insufficiency (Addison's disease) is caused by destruction or atrophy of the adrenal cortex leading to glucocorticoid and mineralocorticoid deficiency. Initiating causes may be unknown (probably immune-mediated), or may result from infectious disease, tumours, infarction or administration of the adrenocorticolytic drug, o,p'-DDD (mitotane). Secondary adrenocortical insufficiency results from inadequate pituitary adrenocorticotrophic hormone (ACTH) production. Circulating glucocorticoid levels are suppressed, while mineralocorticoid production is usually not significantly affected. Iatrogenic secondary adrenocortical insufficiency most often develops following abrupt withdrawal of exogenous corticosteroid or progestogen therapy (Chastain, Graham and Nichols, 1981; Feldman and Peterson, 1984).

Clinical signs in patients with hypoadrenocorticism relate to the degree and duration of glucocorticoid and/or mineralocorticoid deficiency. Endogenous cortisol deficiency may lead to decreased gluconeogenesis and glycogenolysis, gastrointestinal upsets such as vomiting and diarrhoea, impaired ability of the kidneys to excrete a water load, decreased vascular sensitivity to catecholamines and depressed mentation. Mineralocorticoid deficiency (primarily aldosterone) results in renal sodium, chloride, and water loss with potassium and hydrogen ion retention. Typically, patients are acidotic, hyponatraemic and hyperkalaemic, with a sodium : potassium ratio of less than 27 : 1. Clinical findings in hypoadrenocorticoid patients may vary from depression, lethargy and muscle weakness to dehydration, severe bradycardia, weak pulses, circulatory shock and even cardiovascular collapse (Schrader, 1986).

Definitive diagnosis of hypoadrenocorticism is based on demonstration of an inadequate cortisol response to exogenous ACTH administration. Primary and secondary hypoadrenocorticism may be differentiated by measurement of basal ACTH levels. ACTH levels are likely to be elevated in cases of primary adrenocortical insufficiency, while patients with secondary hypoadrenocorticism as a result of pituitary failure are unable to secrete a normal amount of ACTH. Secondary hypoadrenocorticoid patients are also likely to have a normal sodium : potassium ratio since aldosterone secretion is usually unaffected.

Treatment of patients with acute adrenocortical insufficiency should be directed towards restoration of circulating blood volume, correction of hyperkalaemia and hyponatraemia, correction of acidosis and glucocorticoid supplementation. Normal (0.9%) saline is the intravenous fluid of choice. It should be administered initially at a rapid rate of 40–80 ml kg^{-1} h^{-1} to correct volume and sodium deficits. The rate of fluid administration and response of the animal should be monitored closely and fluid rate tapered off quickly once blood volume has been restored as animals with glucocorticoid or mineralocorticoid deficiencies are less able to excrete a normal water load. Intravenous fluids should be supplemented with sodium bicarbonate as needed to correct hyperkalaemia and acidosis. Large doses of a rapidly acting glucocorticoid such as dexamethasone sodium phosphate (2–4 mg kg^{-1}) should be administered to correct endogenous corticosteroid deficits. Additional therapy with a mineralocorticoid agent such as desoxycorticosterone acetate (DOCA: 1–5 mg i.m.) has also been advocated (Schrader, 1986).

Patients with primary adrenocortical insufficiency are normally maintained on oral or depot injection mineralocorticoid therapy. Approximately 50% of dogs will require additional glucocorticoid supplementation. The addition of sodium chloride to the diet has also been suggested (Schrader, 1986). Animals with substantiated secondary hypoadrenocorticism usually do not require mineralocorticoid or sodium chloride supplementation. Glucocorticoid supplementation is usually sufficient in these cases (Schrader, 1986).

Preanaesthetic assessment and preparation. In most cases, the operative procedure is unrelated to the primary endocrinopathy and the patient is stabilized on chronic corticosteroid supplementation. Occasionally, animals are presented for emergency surgery with recently diagnosed, but unstable acute adrenocortical insufficiency. In these cases, the decision to operate is necessarily a compromise between the urgency of the procedure and the condition of the animal. The animal should be stabilized as far as possible before surgery using the therapeutic protocol outlined previously. In any case, anaesthesia should not be induced before normalization of blood volume, correction of electrolyte and acid–base abnormalities and initiation of intravenous glucocorticoid supplementation (Schrader, 1986).

Blood urea nitrogen (BUN), serum electrolytes, packed cell volume (PCV) and total solids (TS) should be determined routinely in all patients with stabilized primary hypoadrenocorticism prior to surgery. If azotaemia, hyponatraemia, hyperkalaemia or dehydration is detected, surgery should be delayed while appropriate intravenous fluid therapy is administered (Peterson, 1987).

Dogs with hyperadrenocorticism which are maintained on o,p'-DDD therapy will have a decreased adrenocortical reserve capacity and therefore require supplemental glucocorticoid therapy during surgery (Peterson, 1984), as outlined below. In addition, although o,p'-DDD therapy usually maintains normal aldosterone secretion, about 5% of dogs will develop iatrogenic hypoadrenocorticism which is characterized by subnormal basal and post-ACTH stimulated cortisol levels, hyperkalaemia and hyponatraemia (Peterson, 1987). These abnormalities should be evaluated in all animals on chronic o,p'-DDD therapy and, if present, should be corrected before surgery.

Abrupt withdrawal of chronic glucocorticoid or progestogen therapy before anaesthesia and surgery in dogs and cats may lead to acute adrenocortical insufficiency (Chastain *et al.*, 1981; Feldman and Peterson, 1984). If feasible, an ACTH stimulation test should be used to evaluate the functional ability of the adrenal cortex in these patients. If this is not possible, then all patients which have received large doses of glucocorticoids or progestogens for longer than a week should receive supplemental glucocorticoids immediately prior to anaesthesia (Peterson, 1987), as outlined below.

Anaesthetic management. Although the majority of patients with adrenocortical insufficiency presented for anaesthesia and surgery will be stabilized on glucocorticoid supplementation, it should be appreciated that the stresses imposed by these procedures will increase the animal's cortisol requirement by five- to tenfold. If this need is not met by additional supplementation, adrenocortical crisis will develop (Dundee, 1957; Weatherill and Spence, 1984).

The dose of glucocorticoid administered should therefore be supraphysiological (5–10 times maintenance) but not excessive or else a delay in wound healing and increase in the incidence of postoperative infections will result (Kehlet, 1975). More importantly, the duration of increased supplementation should be determined by the nature and extent of the surgical procedure (Peterson, 1987). Major surgical procedures will be associated with prolonged stresses requiring glucocorticoid supplementation for at least several days. Animals which undergo minor procedures, however, may only require additional supplementation until the day following surgery.

An appropriate corticosteroid supplementation regimen suggested by Peterson (1987) for use in small animals undergoing major procedures is to administer soluble hydrocortisone (4–5 mg kg^{-1}), dexamethasone (0.1–0.2 mg kg^{-1}) or prednisolone sodium succinate (1–2 mg kg^{-1}) intravenously either 1 hour before anaesthesia or at the time of induction. At the end of the procedure, a similar dose of the agent chosen should be administered either intramuscularly or intravenously. On the next day, supplementation should be continued at five times maintenance dosage as either prednisone (0.5 mg kg^{-1} twice a day), prednisolone (0.5 mg kg^{-1} twice a day), cortisone acetate (2.5 mg kg^{-1} twice a day) or dexamethasone (0.1 mg kg^{-1} once a day). Unless complications develop, the animal can be returned to a normal maintenance glucocorticoid regimen by the third postoperative day. If complications such as infection develop or persist, the dosage of supplemental corticosteroid should be maintained at, or increased to, five times the maintenace level until these problems are resolved.

For animals undergoing minor surgical procedures, a similar regimen is used except that these patients may be returned to a maintenance corticosteroid schedule by the first postoperative day (Peterson, 1987).

There are no specific anaesthetic drug combinations which are indicated for use in patients with adrenocortical insufficiency. In general, anaesthetic agents should be chosen to produce smooth, stress-free induction, maintenance and recovery from anaesthesia (Weatherill and Spence, 1984). Etomidate, a hypnotic induction agent, is contraindicated for use in hypoadrenocorticoid patients because it has been shown to suppress adrenocortical function both in human and canine surgical patients (Wagner and White, 1984; Druse-Elliott, Swanson and Aucoin, 1987). Thiobarbiturates may be more appropriate as intravenous induction agents in these patients. Agents which are hypotensive or cardiac depressant should also be avoided in patients with unstabilized acute adrenocortical insufficiency.

Perioperative stress in unstable glucocorticoid deficient dogs may result in acute cardiovascular collapse characterized by peripheral vasoconstriction, inadequate venous return and cardiac output, and decreased myocardial contractility. The circulatory system should be closely monitored for signs of cardiovascular collapse in such patients both during and following surgery. Such signs may include pale mucous membranes and a weak and thready pulse in conjunction with an increased heart rate. Measurement of arterial blood pressure in these patients is extremely useful. If cardiovascular collapse develops it should be treated by the rapid intravenous administration of a crystalloid solution (normal saline at 40–80 ml kg^{-1} h^{-1}). Colloid solutions (dextran 70 at 20 ml kg^{-1} total dose) and inotropic agents such as dopamine (2–5 μg kg^{-1} min^{-1}) will expand blood volume and improve cardiac performance respectively. A rapidly acting glucocorticoid such as prednisolone sodium succinate (5–10 mg kg^{-1} i.v.) should also be administered at this time.

Close attention should be paid to the patient's fluid, electrolyte and acid–base balance, both during and following surgery, particularly if abnormalities existed before surgery. Abnormalities should be corrected by appropriate intravenous fluid therapy.

Hyperadrenocorticism (Cushing's disease)

Spontaneous hyperadrenocorticism (Cushing's disease) is a common endocrinopathy in middle-aged to older dogs resulting from excessive cortisol production by the adrenal cortex. In 85–95% of affected dogs, hypercortisolaemia is caused by excessive ACTH secretion by the pituitary gland resulting in bilateral adrenocortical hyperplasia. In the remaining 5–15% of cases, unilateral cortisol-secreting tumours of the adrenal cortex are responsible (Peterson, 1986).

Clinical signs in these patients reflect multisystemic dysfunction and are associated with prolonged glucocorticoid excess. Signs related to the compressive effects of adrenal, pituitary tumours or metastases may also contribute to the clinical picture. The most common clinical findings associated with hyperadrenocorticism include polyuria and polydipsia, pendulous abdomen, hepatomegaly, hair loss, polyphagia and muscle weakness. Common clinical pathology abnormalities include a mature leucocytosis with an absolute eosinopenia, and an elevation in alkaline phosphatase activity. Excessive glucocorticoid levels cause induction of the hepatic isoenzyme of alkaline phosphatase (Peterson, 1986).

Diagnosis of hyperadrenocorticism is based on demonstrating an exaggerated response to exogenous ACTH administration or, more reliably, by obtaining no response to the low-dose dexamethasone suppression test (Feldman, 1983a). Differentiation of pituitary-dependent hyperadrenocorticism (PDH) from adrenocortical tumour may then be achieved by determining basal endogenous ACTH levels or, less satisfactorily, by use of the high-dose dexamethasone suppression test (Feldman 1983b). Details of these diagnostic tests are given elsewhere (Peterson, 1984, 1986).

Dogs with PDH can be treated by either bilateral adrenalectomy or hypophysectomy. However, because of the risks associated with these procedures and the need for lifelong hormone replacement therapy, the majority of affected dogs are treated medically with the adrenocorticolytic agent o,p'-DDD (Peterson, 1984). The treatment of choice for dogs with adrenocortical tumour is surgical excision.

Preanaesthetic assessment and preparation. Dogs with uncontrolled hyperadrenocorticism commonly have multisystemic abnormalities which significantly increase the risks of anaesthesia and surgery. Probably the most important of these to the anaesthetist is the effect of chronic hypercortisolaemia on cardiorespiratory function.

Patients with hyperadrenocorticism often have fluid retention and hypertension. These changes frequently occur in association with valvular disease in older dogs and may result in left ventricular hypertrophy and congestive heart failure (Peterson, 1987). Cardiac function should be carefully evaluated in these patients prior to anaesthesia, including auscultation of the chest for murmurs, thoracic radiography to assess heart chamber enlargement, and, if possible, echocardiography. Patients with congestive heart failure will need to be treated with diuretics and inotropic agents before anaesthesia can be contemplated.

Ventilatory function may be compromised in these patients because of respiratory muscle weakness, thoracic fat deposition and restriction of diaphragmatic excursion resulting from hepatomegaly and intra-abdominal fat accumulation (Peterson, 1987). The adequacy of ventilatory function should be assessed preoperatively by measuring arterial blood gases to detect hypercapnia, and if possible, measurement of minute respiratory volume (Dodman *et al.*, 1987). Animals in which ventilatory function is determined to be inadequate will require ventilatory support in the form of intermittent positive pressure ventilation (IPPV) intraoperatively and possibly postoperatively.

It is important to evaluate the volume status and electrolyte and acid–base balance of animals with hyperadrenocorticism before anaesthesia. Excessive blood levels of mineralocorticoids cause sodium and water retention along with depletion of potassium and hydrogen ions. The extent of the resultant overhydration, hypokalaemia and metabolic acidosis should be evaluated preoperatively and intravenous fluid therapy instituted to correct any abnormalities (Peterson, 1986). On the other hand, dogs which have been maintained on *o,p'*-DDD therapy may develop iatrogenic hypoadrenocorticism and can be mineralocorticoid deficient (Peterson, 1984). These dogs will be volume depleted, hyperkalaemic and acidotic, and therefore require different intravenous fluid therapy and glucocorticoid and mineralocorticoid supplementation before anaesthesia.

Diabetes mellitus is often found in association with hyperadrenocorticism (Peterson *et al.*, 1981). Cortisol, and glucocorticoids in general, antagonize the hypoglycaemic effect of insulin. Exogenous insulin requirement in these animals is highly dependent on the circulating level of cortisol (Peterson, Altszuler and Nichols, 1984). Animals that are treated with *o,p'*-DDD require less insulin as the plasma level of cortisol decreases and the cause of insulin resistance is removed (Peterson, 1986). Resection of an adrenal tumour may also significantly decrease the plasma cortisol level and therefore result in a relative hyperinsulinaemia. Fasting blood glucose levels should be evaluated immediately prior to surgery to evaluate the adequacy of the animal's insulin dosage regimen. Repeated measurement of blood glucose throughout surgery and postoperatively is also recommended, particularly in instances when plasma glucocorticoid levels are likely to be changing.

Preoperative use of *o,p'*-DDD or inhibitors of adrenocortical function, such as metyrapone or aminoglutethimide, should be considered in patients with severe, advanced hyperadrenocorticism (Weatherill and Spence, 1984; Peterson, 1987).

Anaesthetic management. The choice of anaesthetic agents for use in patients with hyperadrenocorticism is dependent on the presence of concurrent systemic disease rather than being directly related to the primary endocrine disturbance (Weatherill and Spence, 1984). Although etomidate has been shown to depress adrenocortical function (Kruse-Elliott *et al.*, 1987), its use as an induction agent has not been shown to be of any significant benefit in these patients. In fact, etomidate may be contraindicated in patients undergoing surgical resection of a unilateral adrenal tumour, where depression of residual adrenocortical function in the remaining adrenal gland would be undesirable. Animals with heart failure or ventilatory compromise should be anaesthetized using techniques previously described (Dodman *et al.*, 1987; Seeler *et al.*, 1988).

The adequacy of ventilation should be evaluated intraoperatively for reasons previously described. This should include measurement of minute respiratory volume with a respirometer and determination of arterial blood gas values (Dodman *et al.*, 1987). When MRV is less than 150 ml kg^{-1} or if P_{CO_2} is greater than 60 mmHg, IPPV should be instituted. Ventilatory care should continue into the immediate postoperative period in such patients.

Cardiovascular function should be closely monitored, particularly where there is likely to be a sudden decrease in plasma cortisol levels and the possibility of a subsequent adrenocortical crisis. This may occur in patients undergoing unilateral or bilateral adrenalectomy, or hypophysectomy. As a general rule, these patients should receive supplemental glucocorticoid therapy prior to induction of anaesthesia, as described in the previous section for patients with adrenocortical insufficiency. Postoperatively, these animals will require continued glucocorticoid supplementation either until the remaining adrenal gland resumes functioning, in the case of unilateral adrenalectomy; or for the remainder of the animal's life, in the case of bilateral adrenalectomy or hypophysectomy. Therapy for animals which develop adrenocortical crisis has been described previously.

ADRENAL MEDULLA

Phaeochromocytoma

Phaeochromocytomas are rare, often functional tumours in the dog arising from chromaffin tissue in the adrenal medulla (Wheeler, 1986).

Clinical manifestations in patients with phaeochromocytoma result from excessive production of catecholamines by the tumour. The clinical presentation of these signs, however, tends to be quite variable and episodic because of the variable degree and intermittent nature of catecholamine release. Hypertension and tachycardia appear to occur most consistently. Other less specific signs may include dyspnoea, weakness, tremors, restlessness, polyuria, polydipsia and anorexia. Because the tumour is locally invasive, approximately one-third of cases will have invasion of tumour thrombus into the caudal vena cava. Such animals may show ascites, oedema of the hind legs and distension of the caudal epigastric vessels. Patients may also present with manifestations resulting from the complications of hypertension, such as epistaxis, cardiomyopathy or cerebral vascular accident (Twedt and Wheeler, 1984; Wheeler, 1986).

A diagnosis of phaeochromocytoma is based on demonstration of inappropriate and excessive catecholamine release. This is usually accomplished by detecting abnormally elevated catecholamine metabolites in the urine, usually vanillylmandelic acid. Localization of the tumour can be accomplished by abdominal palpation, if it is large enough, or by plain and contrast radiographic techniques. Non-selective venography of the caudal vena cava will often show invasion of the tumour into this vessel (Wheeler, 1986). Computerized tomography, where available, appears to be the most reliable and safest method for determination of the location and extent of local tumour invasion (Marschall, 1987).

The treatment of choice in patients with phaeochromocytoma is surgical resection (Wheeler, 1986). Medical treatment is usually reserved for stabilization of patients prior to surgery, or for chronic management of animals with inoperable or metastatic tumours. α-Methyltyrosine, a tyrosine hydroxylase inhibitor, has been used to suppress catecholamine synthesis in human patients, but its use is limited to patients with metastatic phaeochromocytoma because of renal and neurological toxicity (Marschall, 1987).

Preanaesthetic assessment and preparation. Adequate preparation is required in these patients in order to avoid serious perioperative complications arising from excessive catecholamine release.

"FURAZOSIN"
"Minipress"

Blood pressure should be normalized before surgery by administration of an α-adrenoceptor blocking agent such as phenoxybenzamine or prazosin. Phenoxybenzamine may be administered at an initial dose of 0.2–0.4 mg kg^{-1} twice a day orally which is gradually increased over several days until hypertension and accompanying signs are no longer apparent. Normally, less than 1.5 mg kg^{-1} twice a day over 10–14 days will normalize blood pressure in most dogs.

β-Adrenoceptor blocking agents such as propranolol may be required in addition to α-blockers for control of cardiac dysrhythmias and tachycardia or for hypertension which persists despite α-adrenoceptor blockade. Relatively low doses of propranolol (0.15–0.5 mg kg^{-1} three times a day orally) are usually required. β-Adrenoceptor blocking drugs must never be given to patients with phaeochromocytoma without α-adrenoceptor blockade or else severe pressor responses may ensue (Wheeler, 1986; Marschall, 1987; Peterson, 1987).

Anaesthetic management. The major objectives involved in formulating an anaesthetic regimen for use in patients with phaeochromocytoma are to avoid provocation of catecholamine release by anaesthetic drugs, to suppress the catecholamine response to surgical stimulation, and to minimize the haemodynamic consequences of tumour handling and removal (Marschall, 1987).

Drugs that release histamine, such as morphine, pethidine and atracurium, should be avoided since histamine is a potent stimulator of catecholamine release (Marschall, 1987). Atropine should not be used in these patients since vagolytic blockade may potentiate the chronotropic and dysrhythmogenic effects of adrenaline (Muir, 1978). Glycopyrrolate may be a better alternative where a reduction in vagal tone is desired. Agents which sensitize the myocardium to catecholamines, such as xylazine and halothane, should also be avoided (Muir, Werner and Hamlin, 1975).

Several drugs have been reported to cause pressor responses in human patients with phaeochromocytoma and are therefore contraindicated for use under these circumstances (Marschall, 1987). Droperidol is thought to cause a pressor response in these patients either directly by stimulating tumour cells or sympathetic nerve endings to release catecholamines, or by inhibiting catecholamine reuptake ino nerve terminals. Other drugs in this category include chlorpromazine, metoclopramide and ephedrine. These drugs should probably be avoided in dogs with phaeochromocytoma.

A satisfactory anaesthetic regimen for the majority of patients with phaeochromocytoma may include premedication with a low dose of acepromazine (0.025–0.05 mg kg^{-1} i.m.), induction with thiopentone (8 mg kg⁻¹ i.v. to effect) and maintenance of anaesthesia with isoflurane. Although acepromazine is chemically related to chlorpromazine, this drug has not been shown to cause an adverse pressor response in patients with phaeochromocytoma. In fact, acepromazine has been recommended for use in these patients because of a number of desirable properties including mild α-adrenoceptor blocking activity and an antidysrhythmic action in the presence of catecholamines (Muir *et al.*, 1975; Peterson, 1987). Blood pressure should be monitored following acepromazine administration and, if hypotension is detected, this should be treated by intravenous infusion of crystalloid solutions. Thiobarbiturates are satisfactory for intravenous induction of anaesthesia in these patients since these drugs do not stimulate catecholamine secretion and minimize the stress response associated with induction (Joyce, Roizen and Eger, 1983). However, in certain instances, these agents may be dysrhythmogenic. As an alternative to the thiobarbiturates, particularly in patients with pre-existent dysrhythmias, an opioid agent such as oxymorphone (0.1–0.2 mg kg⁻¹ i.v.) may be used for induction. Isoflurane, or alternatively methoxyflurane or enflurane, are preferred to halothane for maintenance of anaesthesia, since these agents do not sensitize the myocardium to catecholamine-induced dysrhythmias to such an extent (Desmonts and Marty, 1984; Hull, 1986).

Intraoperative problems which may be encountered in patients with phaeochromocytoma include hypertension, hypovolaemia and cardiac dysrhythmias. Monitoring in these animals should include measurement of arterial pressure, central venous pressure (CVP) and observation of the electrocardiogram with an oscilloscope.

If acute hypertension develops following induction or during manipulation of the tumour, intravenous boluses of a short-acting α-adrenoceptor blocker, such as phentolamine (0.02–1.0 mg kg⁻¹) should be administered (Peterson, 1987). Nitroprusside, a direct acting vasodilator, has also been recommended, and is widely used for this purpose in human patients with phaeochromocytoma (Marschall, 1987). Ventricular dysrhythmias and tachycardia usually respond to small doses of a β-adrenoceptor blocker such as propranolol (0.03–0.1 mg kg⁻¹ i.v.). Alternatively, ventricular dysrhythmias which do not respond to propranolol may be treated with lignocaine boluses (1–2 mg kg⁻¹ i.v.).

Throughout surgery, a balanced electrolyte solution such as lactated Ringer's solution should be infused to maintain a normal CVP. A rapid fall in arterial pressure may occur following tumour resection associated with a reduction in peripheral vascular tone. These tumours commonly involve the caudal vena cava; therefore significant blood loss may also occur at this time. These events should be treated by rapid intravenous infusion of a crystalloid solution. Colloid solutions such as dextran 70 are also efficacious. The CVP should be used to estimate the correct fluid administration rate and to avoid overtransfusion.

Postoperatively, measurement of both arterial pressure and CVP should continue until values return to normal. It is not uncommon for many patients to have mild, but transient, hypertension for the first 24 hours following surgery (Peterson, 1987). Sustained hypertension may indicate the presence of metastatic tumour.

THYROID

Hypothyroidism

Hypothyroidism has been reported to be the most common endocrinopathy in the dog (Rosychuk, 1986). Most cases have an early age of onset (2–5 years) and result from a primary disease of the thyroid gland (Fraser and Mays, 1986). Feline hypothyroidism is extremely rare, but may develop following surgical or radioisotope treatment for hyperthyroidism (Peterson and Turrel, 1986).

Clinical signs are the result of a reduction in basal metabolic rate. Affected animals commonly show lethargy, a reduction in exercise tolerance, hypothermia, bradycardia, a mild to moderate anaemia, slight to marked obesity and characteristic dermatological abnormalities (Fraser and Mays, 1986).

Diagnosis is based on demonstrating decreased levels of circulating thyroid hormones, including thyroxine (T_4) and triiodothyronine (T_3). A thyroid-stimulating hormone (TSH) response test may be required in equivocal cases (Fraser and Mays, 1986).

Hypothyroid animals are normally treated with L-thyroxine until thyroxine levels return to normal. Marked improvement in the animal's condition usually occurs within 10–14 days; however, complete recovery may take several months (Fraser and Mays, 1986).

Preanaesthetic assessment and preparation. Considering the depression of physiological function in these animals and the likelihood of increased sensitivity to normal doses of anaesthetic agents, elective surgery should be delayed until a euthyroid state has been achieved (Murkin, 1982). L-Thyroxine (20 μg kg^{-1} daily) should be administered for at least 2 weeks, at which time the anaesthetic risks are reduced to those of animals without thyroid disease (Peterson, 1987).

If emergency surgery is indicated, it is possible to replenish the animal's thyroid hormone levels rapidly using a single intravenous dose of L-thyroxine (20–40 μg kg^{-1}) or alternatively by administering an oral dose of a rapidly acting thyroid hormone such as

L-triiodothyronine at a dose of 4–6 μg kg⁻¹ four times a day (Peterson, 1987). Circulating thyroid hormone levels are usually significantly increased within several hours following initiation of therapy; however, it should be appreciated that there is a risk of inducing thyrotoxicosis with this approach.

Anaesthetic management. Important abnormalities in relation to anaesthesia that accompany hypothyroidism include thermoregulation abnormalities (hypothermia), decreased myocardial contractility, sinus bradycardia, decreased drug metabolism and obesity (Rosychuk, 1986). Careful selection of anaesthetic agents and reduced drug dosages will be required in thyroid hormone deficient animals to avoid profound and prolonged physiological depression.

Hypothyroid animals are likely to be mentally depressed by virtue of their disease and may not require sedative premedication. Opioid agents, such as butorphanol (0.05–0.1 mg kg⁻¹ i.m.) or pethidine (3–5 mg kg⁻¹ i.m.) may be administered before anaesthesia to provide some sedation, reduce the required doses of induction and maintenance agents and supplement analgesia (Dodman, Seeler and Court, 1984). An anticholinergic agent such as atropine (0.02–0.06 mg kg⁻¹ i.m.) should be used in combination with these agents to avoid bradydysrhythmias. Phenothiazine derivatives, such as acepromazine, should not be used in these animals because of the risks of prolonged sedation, hypotension and hypothermia associated with its vasodilatory effects.

Cardiac output and myocardial reserve are reduced in hypothyroid animals (Rosychuk, 1986). Minimal doses of intravenous induction agents, like the thiobarbiturates, should be used in these patients to avoid further cardiovascular depression. A safer alternative would be to induce anaesthesia with an inhalational agent such as halothane or isoflurane which would allow rapid reversal of any untoward changes. Halothane may be a better maintenance agent than isoflurane for use in hypothyroid patients since it causes less peripheral vasodilatation (Hickey and Eger, 1986) and therefore might be associated with less heat loss. On the other hand, isoflurane is a better agent for use in patients with significant myocardial depression (Hickey and Eger, 1986).

Hypothyroid animals are predisposed to hypotension and hypothermia. Arterial pressure and core body temperature should be monitored in these animals, and any abnormalities corrected. Hypothermia may be prevented and, if necessary, treated by using warmed intravenous fluids, a circulating warm water blanket, hot water bottles and a radiant heat lamp (Dodman *et al.*, 1984).

Ventilatory function is readily depressed by anaesthetic agents. An increased sensitivity to anaesthetic agents coupled with restrictions to ventilation imposed by obesity may lead to ventilatory failure in anaesthetized hypothyroid patients. Ventilatory function should be assessed in these animals by measurement of MRV or arterial blood gases, and if ventilation is found to be inadequate, IPPV should be instituted.

Postoperatively, a prolonged recovery from anaesthesia compared with normal animals should be anticipated. Fluid balance and body temperature should be closely monitored during this time.

Hyperthyroidism

Hyperthyroidism (thyrotoxicosis) is an endocrine disorder resulting from excessive circulating levels of the thyroid hormones, thyroxine (T_4) and triiodothyronine (T_3) (Peterson and Turrel, 1986). This disease occurs most commonly in middle-aged to older cats, but also develops rarely in the dog. Idiopathic functional thyroid adenoma involving one or both thyroid lobes is the commonest cause of feline hyperthyroidism, while thyroid carcinoma is the primary cause of hyperthyroidism in the dog (Fraser and Mays, 1986).

Hyperthyroidism causes multisystemic disorders associated with a thyrotoxic hypermetabolic state. Common clinical signs include weight loss, hyperexcitability, polyphagia and tachycardia. Polyuria, polydipsia, vomiting and cardiac murmurs are also frequently observed. Palpable enlargement of one or both of the thyroid lobes is usually detectable in 85–90% of cats with hyperthyroidism. Many cats in which thyroid gland enlargement is not palpable have affected lobes that have descended into the thoracic cavity (Peterson and Turrel, 1986).

Definitive diagnosis of this condition is based on demonstrating abnormally elevated circulating thyroid hormone concentrations (Peterson, 1986). Thyroid scintigraphic imaging is an extremely useful diagnostic tool which aids in determining the extent of thyroid involvement (either unilateral or bilateral), localizes ectopic thyroids and helps identify the presence of metastatic disease (Peterson and Becker, 1984).

Feline hyperthyroidism can be treated in a number of ways. Surgical thyroidectomy or radiotherapy with ^{131}I provides permanent remission, while chemotherapy with the antithyroid drugs, propylthiouracil (PTU) or methimazole, is usually reserved for temporary control before definitive surgical treatment.

Preanaesthetic assessment and preparation. Abnormalities related to thyrotoxicosis which should be evaluated before anaesthesia include hypertrophic cardiomyopathy, heart murmurs, tachycardia and cardiac dysrhythmias (Peterson *et al.*, 1983). Congestive heart failure may occur in 15% of hyperthyroid cats (Peterson, 1986). The chest should be auscultated for murmurs or gallop rhythms. An elecrocardiogram should be taken to identify and quantify rhythm disturbances. Thoracic radiographs and, if possible, echocardiography should be used to detect and qualify heart chamber enlargement. Fortunately, the majority of these changes will resolve with effective antithyroid therapy. It is important to identify animals with congestive heart failure since they will require additional therapy with diuretics and positive inotropic agents before anaesthesia.

Polyuria, polydipsia and an increase in the activity of the serum liver enzymes alanine aminotransferase (ALT), aspartate aminotransferase (AST) and alkaline phosphatase (AP) are commonly detected in hyperthyroid cats (Peterson, 1986). The cause of these changes is largely unknown; however, they are not usually indicative of significant renal or hepatic disease. On the other hand, the persistence of these signs following antithyroid therapy may indicate concurrent, but unrelated, organic disease which will require further investigation.

All hyperthyroid animals should be treated with one of the antithyroid drugs before thyroidectomy, or before any other elective procedure requiring anaesthesia, in order to achieve a euthyroid state. This will effectively resolve many of the abnormalities associated with thyrotoxicosis and therefore significantly decrease the risks associated with anaesthesia in these animals (Peterson, 1987). Methimazole (1 mg kg^{-1} three times a day) is the drug of choice because of a lower incidence of side effects compared with PTU (Peterson, Kintzer and Hurvitz, 1985). Serious reactions such as agranulocytosis and severe thrombocytopenia can still occur in a small percentage of cats treated with methimazole, necessitating periodic haematological screening.

Serum levels of the thyroid hormones will usually return to normal levels within 2 weeks of treatment with methimazole (Peterson et al., 1985). If this does not occur, the dose can be increased to 1.5 mg kg^{-1} three times a day. Most systemic dysfunctions will significantly improve or resolve in 2–3 weeks following establishment of a euthyroid state. Occasionally, methimazole therapy may be ineffective or the animal may develop adverse side effects necessitating termination of therapy. In these instances, propranolol, a β-adrenoceptor antagonist, may be used to control tachydysrhythmias and hyperexcitability before anaesthesia (Peterson, 1987). The recommended dosage regimen is 0.5–1.0 mg kg^{-1} three times a day for 7–14 days. Propranolol should be used cautiously in cats with congestive heart failure because of its negative inotropic effects.

Anaesthetic management. Most routine anaesthetic regimens are safe for use in these patients, provided a euthyroid state has been attained for at least 2 weeks before anaesthesia. Animals in which this has not been achieved will require special consideration both in the selection of anaesthetic agents and in the attention given to intraoperative complications.

Anaesthetic agents which increase catecholamine release (such as ketamine or tiletamine), decrease vagal tone (such as atropine) or increase myocardial sensitivity to the dysrhythmogenic effects of catecholamines (such as halothane or xylazine) should be avoided in unstabilized hyperthyroid animals.

Acepromazine (0.05–1.0 mg kg^{-1} i.m.) is a useful premedicant in these animals because it produces good sedation, thereby decreasing perioperative stress, and has been shown to decrease the incidence of dysrhythmias induced by thiobarbiturates and inhalational agents (Muir *et al.*, 1975). If an anticholinergic agent is required to prevent or treat an elevation in vagal tone, such as when an opioid agent is used, glycopyrrolate is preferable to atropine because this agent has a minimal effect on cardiac rate and rhythm (Short and Miller, 1978).

Intravenous induction of anaesthesia is preferred to inhalational induction, except in depressed patients, because of the risk of catecholamine release associated with struggling during mask induction. Hyperthyroid cats tend to be hyperexcitable and do not readily accept inhalational induction techniques. Thiobarbiturates are satisfactory induction agents in hyperthyroid animals because they possess antithyroid actvity and do not cause catecholamine release (Stehling, 1974; Joyce *et al.*, 1983). They do, however, sensitize the heart to the dysrhythmogenic effects of catecholamines. The combination steroid anaesthetic, alphaxalone/alphadolone, may be the intravenous induction agent of choice in the hyperthyroid cat since it has been shown to reduce the incidence of catecholamine-induced dysrhythmias in this species (Dodds and Twissel, 1972).

Isoflurane is preferable to halothane or methoxyflurane for maintenance of anaesthesia in hyperthyroid patients. Isoflurane does not sensitize the heart to catecholamines, produces minimal myocardial depression, and possesses a low blood solubility allowing rapid recovery from anaesthesia should intraoperative problems arise (Hickey and Eger, 1986).

Heart rate and rhythm should be monitored continuously throughout surgery using an electrocardiographic oscilloscope. Ventricular dysrhythmias are common, particularly in animals which were not rendered euthyroid before anaesthesia (Peterson, 1987). Such dysrhythmias usually respond to small doses of propranolol (0.01–0.05 mg kg^{-1} i.v.) or lignocaine (0.5–1 mg kg^{-1} i.v.).

Warmth should be provided during recovery from anaesthesia

particularly in hyperthyroid cats which tend to be thin and lose body heat readily. Some form of oxygen supplementation should also be used during recovery. Hyperthyroid animals usually have higher metabolic oxygen demand than euthyroid animals and are therefore prone to hypoxia and related complications.

Postoperative complications related to thyroidectomy may include iatrogenic hypoparathyroidism, Horner's syndrome and vocal cord paralysis (Birchard, Peterson and Jacobson, 1984).

Although attempts are usually made to preserve the external parathyroid glands, bilateral thyroidectomy may result in iatrogenic hypoparathyroidism and subsequent to this, hypocalcaemia. Serum calcium should be monitored for at least 3 days in these patients (Peterson, 1987). Therapy with intravenous calcium and vitamin D is indicated if the serum calcium decreases in conjunction with clinical signs of hypocalcaemia, such as muscle tremors, tetany or convulsions. Thyroid hormone replacement therapy should also be initiated in these animals 24–48 hours following total thyroidectomy (Peterson, 1987).

REFERENCES

Ammon, J. R. (1987). *38th Annual Refresher Course of the ASA*, 272.

Bevan, D. R. (1980). In *General Anaesthesia*, eds. T. C. Gray, J. F. Nunn & J. E. Utting, 4th edn, p. 1017. London: Butterworths.

Birchard, S. J., Peterson, M. E. and Jacobson, A. (1984). *Journal of the American Animal Hospital Association* **20**, 705.

Booth, N. H. (1982). In *Veterinary Pharmacology and Therapeutics*, eds. N. H. Booth & L. E. McDonald, 5th edn, p. 297. Ames, Iowa: Iowa State University Press.

Brock, K. B. (1983). *Proceedings of the Refresher Courses in Anaesthesia and Intensive Care* **62**, 235.

Chastain, C. B. (1981). *Journal of the American Veterinary Medical Association* **179**, 972.

Chastain, C. B., Graham, C. L. and Nichols, C. E. (1981). *American Journal of Veterinary Research* **42**, 2029.

Clarke, C. S. J. (1970). *British Journal of Anaesthesia* **42**, 45.

Desmonts, J. M. and Marty, J. (1984). *British Journal of Anaesthesia* **56**, 781.

Dodds, M. G. and Twissell, D. J. (1972). *Postgraduate Medical Journal* **48** (suppl. 2), 17.

Dodman, N. H., Seeler, D. C. and Court, M. H. (1984). *British Veterinary Journal* **140**, 505.

Dodman, N. H., Seeler, D. C., Norman, W. M. and Court, M. H. (1987). *British Veterinary Journal* **143**, 291.

Dundee, J. W. (1957). *British Journal of Anaesthesia* **29**, 166.

Eigenman, J. E. (1981). *Journal of the American Animal Hospital Association* **17**, 805.

Ewart, R. B., Rusy, B. F. and Bradford, M. W. (1981). *Anesthesia and Analgesia* **60**, 878.

Feldman, E. C. (1983a). *Journal of the American Veterinary Medical Association* **182**, 506.

Feldman, E. C. (1983b). *Journal of the American Veterinary Medical Association* **183**, 195.

Feldman, E. C. and Nelson, R. W. (1986). In *Current Veterinary Therapy IX. Small Animal Practice*, ed. R. W. Kirk, p. 1000. Philadelphia: W. B. Saunders Co.

Feldman, E. C. and Peterson, M. E. (1984). *Veterinary Clinics of North America (Small Animal Practice)* **14(4)**, 751.

Fraser, C. M. and Mays, A. M. (1986). In *The Merck Veterinary Manual*, 6th edn. p. 246. Rahway, New Jersey: Merck and Co., Inc.

Gingevich, R., Wright, P. H. and Paradise, R. R. (1980). *Anesthesiology* **53**, 219.

Hardie, E. M., Rawlings, C.A. and George, J. W. (1985). *American Journal of Veterinary Research* **46**, 1700.

Hickey, R. F. and Eger, E. I. (1986). In *Anesthesia*, ed. R. D. Miller, 2nd edn, p. 649. New York: Churchill Livingstone.

Higgins, G. A. (1979). *Surgical Clinics of North America* **59**, 131.

Hsu, W. H. and Hembrough, F. B. (1982). *American Journal of Veterinary Research* **43**, 2060.

Hull, C. J. (1986). *British Journal of Anaesthesia* **58**, 1453.

Joyce, J. T., Roizen, M. F. and Eger, E. I. (1983). *Anesthesiology* **59**, 19.

Kehlet, H. (1975). *Acta Anaesthesiologica Scandinavica* **19**, 260.

Kraegen, E. W., Lazarus, L., Meler, H., Campbell, L. and Chia, Y. O. (1975). *British Medical Journal* **iii**, 463.

Kruse-Elliott, K. T., Swanson, C. R. and Aucoin, D. P. (1987). *American Journal of Veterinary Research* **48(7)**, 1098.

Leifer, C. E. (1986). In *Current Veterinary Therapy IX, Small Animal Practice*, ed. R. W. Kirk, p. 982. Philadelphia: W. B. Saunders Co.

Leifer, C. E. and Peterson, M. E. (1984). *Veterinary Clinics of North America (Small Animal Practice)* **14**, 873.

Leifer, C. E. Peterson, M. E. and Matus, R. E. (1986). *Journal of the American Veterinary Medical Association* **188**, 60.

Marschall, K. E. (1987). *38th Annual Refresher Courses of the ASA*, 154.

Mehlhaff, C. J., Peterson, M. E., Patnaik, A. K., *et al.* (1985). *Journal of the American Animal Hospital Association* **21**, 607.

Muir, J. J., Endres, S. M., Offord, K., Van Heerden, J. A. and Tinker, J. H. (1983). *Anesthesiology* **59**, 511.

Muir, W. W. (1978). *Journal of the American Veterinary Medical Association* **172**, 917.

Muir, W. W., Werner, L. L. and Hamlin, R. L. (1975). *American Journal of Veterinary Research* **36**, 1299.

Murkin, J. M. (1982). *Anesthesia and Analgesia* **61**, 371.

Nelson, R. W. and Feldman, E. C. (1986). In *Current Veterinary Therapy IX, Small Animal Practice*, ed. R. W. Kirk, p. 991. Philadelphia: W. B. Saunders Co.

Peterson, M. E. (1984). *Veterinary Clinics of North America (Small Animal Practice)* **14**, 731.

Peterson, M. E. (1986). In *Current Veterinary Therapy IX, Small Animal Practice*, ed. R. W. Kirk, p. 963. Philadelphia: W. B. Saunders Co.

Peterson, M. E. (1987). In *Principles and Practice of Veterinary Anesthesia*, ed. C. E. Short, p. 251. Phildelphia: W. B. Saunders Co.

Peterson, M. E., and Becker, D. V. (1984). *Veterinary Radiology* **25**, 23.

Peterson, M. E. and Turrel, J. M. (1986). In *Current Veterinary Therapy IX, Small Animal Practice*, ed. R. W. Kirk, p. 1026. Philadelphia: W. B. Saunders Co.

Peterson, M. E., Birchard, S.J. and Mehlhaff, C. J. (1984). *Veterinary Clinics of North America (Small Animal Practice)* **14(4)**, 911.

Peterson, M. E., Kintzer, P. P. and Hurvitz, A. I. (1985). *Proceedings of the American College of Veterinary Internal Medicine* p. 128.

Peterson, M. E., Nesbitt, G. H. and Schaer. M. (1981). *Journal of the American Veterinary Medical Association* **178**, 66.

Peterson, M. E., Kintzer, P. P., Cavanagh, P. G., Fox, P. R., *et al.* (1983). *Journal of the American Veterinary Medical Association* **183**, 103.

Petty, C. and Cunningham, N. L. (1974). *Anesthesiology* **40**, 400.

Pulver, J. J., Cullen, B. F., Miller, D.R. and Valenta, L. J. (1980). *Anesthesia and Analgesia* **59**, 950.

Rosychuk, R. (1986). In *Current Veterinary Therapy IX, Small Animal Practice*, ed. R. W. Kirk, p. 869. Philadelphia: W. B. Saunders Co.

Schrader, L. A. (1986). In *Current Veterinary Therapy IX, Small Animal Practice*, ed. R. W. Kirk, p. 972. Philadelphia: W. B. Saunders Co.

Seeler, D. C., Dodman, N. H., Norman, W. M. and Court, M. H. (1988). *British Veterinary Journal* **144**, 108.

Short, C. E. and Miller, R. L. (1978). *Veterinary Medicine and Small Animal Clinician* **73**, 1269.

Stehling, L. C. (1974). *Anesthesiology* **41**, 585.

Suffecol, S. L. (1980). In *Anesthesia and the Patient with Endocrine*

Disease, eds. B. R. Brown, D. C. Blitt & A. H. Gieseche, p. 11. Philadelphia: F. A. Davis.

Twedt, D. C. and Wheeler, S. L. (1984). *Veterinary Clinics of North America (Small Animal Practice)* **14**, 767.

van Heerden, J. A., Edis, A. J. and Service, F. J. (1979). *Annals of Surgery* **189**, 677.

Wagner, R. L. and White, P. F. (1984). *Anesthesiology* **61**, 647.

Weatherill, D. and Spence, A. A. (1984). *British Journal of Anaesthesia* **56**, 741.

Wheeler, S. L. (1986). In *Current Veterinary Therapy IX, Small Animal Practice*, ed. R. W. Kirk, p. 977. Philadelphia: W. B. Saunders Co.

Winegrad, A. I. (1986), *Diabetes* **36**, 396.

10

Anaesthesia for patients with central nervous system disease: general considerations

General anaesthesia is invariably required for the surgical management of diseases of the central nervous system (CNS) in small animal patients. Many neurodiagnostic procedures such as collection of cerebrospinal fluid, contrast radiography, and computed tomography also require a motionless patient. By the nature of their action, general anaesthetics alter normal neural electrical activity and blood supply. In patients with CNS disease, where either electrophysiological function, blood flow regulation or both are abnormal, the interaction of general anaesthetics and CNS function is often adversely exaggerated. Optimizing the anaesthetic technique in these patients to minimize these effects can have a marked impact on neurological outcome.

The chapter examines two common manifestations of CNS disease: *intracranial hypertension* and *seizures*. The changes in normal physiology, interactions with anaesthetic agents and techniques, and management of these manifestations are discussed.

ANAESTHESIA AND INTRACRANIAL HYPERTENSION

Intracranial blood flow

The brain is a highly vascular organ receiving some 20% of the cardiac output (Shapiro, 1986a). This high blood flow is required to meet the brain's metabolic requirements which are a consequence of extensive electrophysiological and cellular homeostatic activities. Intrinsic and extrinsic factors modulate regional and global cerebral blood flow (CBF) such that under normal circumstances a satisfactory metabolic demand to substrate supply relationship is maintained.

Intrinsic regulation of CBF is a complicated process which is far from understood. Although it is known that local metabolic factors play a major role in influencing the rate and distribution of CBF, the exact coupling mechanism of metabolism to blood flow is unknown (Shapiro, 1986a). Implicated modulators of local blood flow include the concentration of extracellular ions (hydrogen, potassium and calcium), the cyclo-oxygenase products of phospholipid metabolism (thromboxane and certain prostaglandins), and adenosine (Kuschinsky and Wahl, 1978; Siesjo, 1984).

There also appear to be neurogenic and myogenic factors involved in the local regulation of CBF (Shapiro, 1986a). The cerebral vasculature, particularly larger vessels, are extensively innervated suggesting that neurogenic mechanisms may be involved in the control of CBF. Myogenic responses of cerebral vascular smooth muscle involve rapid compensatory changes in vessel diameter in response to alterations in perfusion pressure. This effect is thought to contribute to some extent to the CBF autoregulatory response. The myogenic response appears to be an intrinsic characteristic of cerebral vessels since it occurs independently of detectable changes in brain metabolites or extracellular ion concentrations (Vinall and Simeone, 1981).

The major extrinsic influences on CBF are cerebral perfusion pressure (CPP), which is the difference between arterial blood pressure and intracranial pressure (ICP), and arterial blood gas tensions ($Paco_2$ and Pao_2). Cerebral blood flow is normally maintained relatively constant at approximately 50 ml 100 g^{-1} min^{-1} between arterial blood pressures of 50 mmHg and 150 mmHg (Fig. 1). This intrinsic property of the cerebral circulation to alter vessel resistance in response to changes in CPP is known as autoregulation (Shapiro, 1986a). Cerebral autoregulation is affected by disease states, volatile anaesthetics and other ceebral vasodilators. Fig. 2 demonstrates the effect of increasing concentrations of volatile anaesthetics on CBF autoregulation.

Cerebral blood flow varies directly with $Paco_2$ and inversely with Pao_2 (Fig 1). Within the physiological range for $Paco_2$, CBF changes about 2 ml 100 g^{-1} min^{-1} for each 1 mmHg change in $Paco_2$. Acute alveolar hyperventilation to a $Paco_2$ of 20 mmHg or less could reduce CBF to the point where ischaemia may occur (Shapiro, 1986a). Oxygen has its greatest influence on CBF when the $Paco_2$ is below the normal physiological limits. When the Pao_2 falls below 50 mmHg, CBF rapidly increases (Shapiro, 1986a). Changes in Pao_2 from 50 mmHg to over 300 mmHg have little effect on CBF.

Pathophysiology of intracranial hypertension

Elevated ICP is the common result of numerous cerebral insults such as head trauma, cerebral ischaemia, infection, tumour and

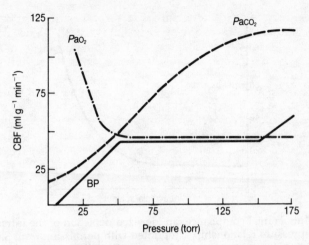

Fig. 1 The influence of alterations in $Paco_2$, Pao_2, and blood pressure (BP) on cerebral blood flow (CBF). (Reprinted with permission from Shapiro, H. M. (1986). In *Anesthesia*, 2nd edn, ed. R. D. Miller, p. 1258. New York: Churchill Livingstone.)

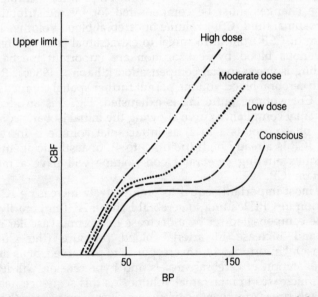

Fig. 2 Representation of the effect of a progressively increased dose of a typical volatile anaesthetic agent on cerebral blood flow (CBF) autoregulation. Both upper and lower thresholds are shifted to the left. (Reprinted with permission from Shapiro, H. M. (1986). In *Anesthesia*, 2nd edn, ed. R. D. Miller, p. 1263. New York: Churchill Livingstone.)

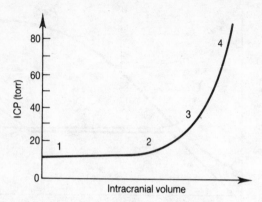

Fig. 3 Intracranial compliance: an idealized depiction of the intracranial volume–pressure relationship. (Reprinted with permission from Shapiro, H. M. (1986). In *Anesthesia*, 2nd edn, ed. R. D. Miller, p. 1566. New York: Churchill Livingstone.)

hydrocephalus (Oliver and Lorenz, 1987; Shapiro, 1986b). Since intracranial structures are virtually incompressible, intracranial volume changes must be compensated for by redistribution of cerebrospinal fluid (CSF) volume or cerebral blood volume. Translocation of CSF from intracranial to extracranial storage sites and into venous blood by reabsorption are important mechanisms providing isobaric spatial compensation (Shapiro, 1986b). Reductions in cerebral blood volume permit further spatial compensation when CSF volume buffering is exhausted. Fig. 3 is an idealized intracranial compliance curve showing the initial isobaric compensation phase (points 1 to 2) as intracranial volume is increased. When ICP is already high (points 3 to 4), anaesthetic agents and techniques altering cerebral blood volume will have a marked impact on ICP.

The most important sequel to progressively increasing ICP is a reduction in CPP leading to cerebral ischaemia. Temporarily, this may be compensated for by a decrease in cerebral vascular resistance and increase in arterial blood pressure (the Cushing response). Unfortunately, this response to preserve CBF is limited since dilatation of cerebral vessels and hypertension will lead to further increases in intacranial volume. As this sequence nears an end stage, areas of ischaemic tissue which contain vessels that lack autoregulatory ability enlarge, such that CBF becomes more directly related to blood pressure. A vicious circle develops such that small decreases in blood pressure may result in regional or total cerebral ischaemia, while increases in blood pressure promote

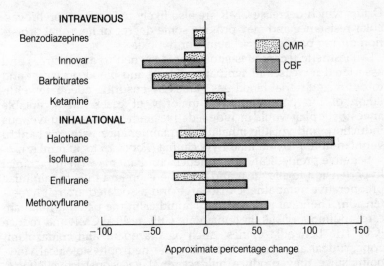

Fig. 4 The relative effects of intravenous and inhalational anaesthetics on cerebral metabolic rate (CMR) and cerebral blood flow (CBF).

oedema formation and further elevate ICP. Global cerebral ischaemia is the ultimate outcome of this process (Shapiro, 1986b).

Clinical signs of intracranial hypertension

Signs resulting from elevations in ICP are relatively non-specific. These may include depressed mentation, behavioural changes, head pressing, pacing and papilloedema (LeCouteur and Turrel, 1986). Changes in the level of consciousness and irregular ventilatory patterns indicate severe increases in ICP. When indicated, CSF pressure measurement may be used to substantiate these findings, but risks brain herniation. The only clinical signs which may be apparent in the comatose or anaesthetized patient are arterial hypertension, bradydysrhythmias and irregular breathing (Shapiro, 1986a).

Anaesthesia and intracranial hypertension

Anaesthetic agents should be selected which increase cerebrovascular resistance, or at least do not promote cerebral vasodilatation, and reduce the cerebral metabolic rate (CMR). Fig. 4 shows the relative effects of selected anaesthetic agents on CBF and CMR. Paradoxically, in patients with elevated ICP, an increase in cerebrovascular resistance can often increase CBF by reducing the cerebral blood volume and ICP and therefore increase the CPP.

Drugs which decrease CMR are also likely to increase cerebrovascular resistance and may provide some degree of neuronal protection during periods of ischaemia or hypoxia.

Anaesthetic techniques should be designed to avoid stress and associated increases in sympathetic tone and blood pressure, and to optimize arterial blood gas values by ensuring adequate ventilation of the patient. In the majority of cases, an acceptable anaesthetic plan would include sedative premedication, intravenous induction, and volatile inhalational maintenance with mechanical ventilation to provide mild hypocapnia ($Poco_2$ 25 to 30 mmHg).

Sedative premedication is beneficial for patients with intracranial hypertension to allay fear and apprehension and thus to minimize preoperative sympathetic discharge and associated arterial hypertension. The ideal premedicant should calm the patient, maintain cardiopulmonary stability, maintain CBF, reduce CMR and reduce ICP. The benzodiazepines, such as diazepam and midazolam, appear ideal as premedicants from the neurophysiological viewpoint since they produce mild cerebral vasoconstrictive effects, decrease CMR and are effective anticonvulsants (Maekawa, Sakabe & Takeshita, 1974). Unfortunately these agents are unreliable as sedatives when used alone in the alert small animal patient, occasionally producing paradoxical excitement. As a result, benzodiazepines are usually reserved for use in the neurologically obtunded patient or are combined with other sedative agents. Low doses of opioid agents have minimal effects on CBF and CMR in small animals (McPherson and Traystman, 1984; Takeshita, Michenfelder and Theye, 1972). Combinations of opioid agents and sedatives, such as fentanyl and droperidol (Innovar Vet) or butorphanol and midazolam, may be efficacious for premedication of fractious animals.

Agents which cause respiratory depression, such as the opioid agents in high doses, should be avoided since hypercapnia will significantly increase ICP. The phenothiazines are also unsuitable for these patients since they lower systemic blood pressure and therefore decrease CPP. The cyclohexamines, such as ketamine and tiletamine, should not be used in patients with intracranial hypertension, since they cause pronounced cerebral vasodilatation, increase CMR and substantially increase ICP. It has been suggested that the cerebral vasodilatation caused by ketamine may be a result of increased regional neuronal activity (Hougaard, Hansen and Broderson, 1974). Although sedative premedicants are useful, they should only be used when considered necessary to promote smooth handling of the patient.

Smooth induction of anaesthesia is highly desirable in patients with increased ICP, and in this respect, induction with an intravenous anaesthetic is ideal. Barbiturates are useful as they cause dose-dependent cerebral vasoconstriction and reduce CMR, thereby reducing ICP and increasing CPP (Pierce, Lambertsen and Deutch, 1962). Provided hypercapnia is avoided, thiopentone appears to be a satisfactory induction agent. Methohexitone is less desirable because of its potential for precipitating seizures with a resultant increase in CMR and cerebral vasodilatation (Ford, Morrell and Whisler, 1982; Wauquier et al., 1978). Alphaxalone/alphadolone (Saffan) is useful for intravenous induction of anaesthesia in cats with increased ICP since this steroid mixture causes a marked decrease in CMR with associated cerebral vasoconstriction and fall in ICP (Pickerodt et al., 1972). Large doses of Saffan should be avoided since this may induce systemic hypotension and cerebral vasodilatation related to histamine release.

At normocapnia, the volatile inhalational anaesthetics, halothane, methoxyflurane and enflurane, increase ICP by cerebral vasodilatation (Campkin and Turner, 1980). This effect may be minimized if moderate hypocapnia is induced by hyperventilation of the patient (Misfeldt, Jorgensen and Spotoft, 1976). However, increases in ICP may still occur, even under these circumstances, in patients with severely elevated pressure (Fitch, Burke and McDowall, 1969). Even nitrous oxide cannot be exempt from such caveats as it has been shown to cause a significant increase in ICP in dogs (Sakabe, Kuramoto and Kumagae, 1976). Enflurane also has the added disadvantage of precipitating seizure activity in the anaesthetized patient thereby adversely increasing CMR (Michenfelder and Cucchiaria, 1974). Isoflurane appears to be the most appropriate inhalational anaesthetic agent when the ICP is elevated. At 1 MAC (minimum alveolar concentration of an inhalational anaesthetic which is required to prevent purposeful movement in response to a noxious stimulus in 50% of a group of test subjects), isoflurane causes minimal increase in CBF in normal patients, while simultaneous hyperventilation of the patient during administration of this agent will produce a stable ICP even in the face of severely decreased intracranial compliance (Tabbador, 1986).

Management of intracranial hypertension

The most important goals in the management of the anaesthetized patient with increased ICP are to maintain cerebral perfusion and arterial oxygenation as near to normal as possible. In this context, it is necessary to reduce ICP to acceptable levels, stabilize arterial blood pressure and optimize arterial blood gas values. Definitive therapy is determined by the aetiological factors(s) causing elevation in ICP. Table 1 lists specific treatment options for the various causes of intracranial hypertension.

Increased ICP resulting from cerebral oedema may be treated by

Table 1. Aetiology and specific therapy for intracranial hypertension

Aetiology	Treatment	Time to response
Cerebral oedema	Fluid restriction	
	Diuretics:	
	osmotic (e.g. mannitol)	15–60 min
	loop (e.g. frusemide)	15–120 min
	Corticosteroids	Hours to days
	Hyperventilation	Immediate
	Cerebral vasoconstrictors	Immediate
Increased cerebral blood volume	Positional change	Immediate
	Stabilize blood pressure	Immediate
	Cerebral vasoconstrictors	Immediate
CSF retention (e.g. hydrocephalus)	Acetazolamide	Hours to days
	Osmotic agents	Hours
	Surgery	Immediate
Intracranial mass	Surgery	Immediate

fluid restriction, the judicious use of diuretics, corticosteroids and by hyperventilation. Fluid restrictions to one-third to one-half of maintenance requirements (30–40 ml kg^{-1} daily) will reduce ICP over a period of days, but should be used with caution in patients in which maintenance of an adequate blood volume is critical. The change in ICP with this method would be too slow to use intraoperatively but may be considered as part of the preoperative preparation of a patient with intracranial hypertension.

More rapid correction of cerebral oedema is achieved through the use of diuretics (Shapiro, 1986b). Mannitol, an osmotic diuretic, is the mainstay of therapy, effecting initial intracranial decompression by osmotic withdrawal of brain water into the intravascular compartment within 10 to 15 minutes of administration. Renal excretion of mannitol occurs within 30 minutes causing systemic dehydration which maintains the reduction in ICP. Deleterious side effects of mannitol include transient intravascular hypervolaemia and exacerbation of CNS lesions with an incomplete blood-brain barrier. Electrolyte depletion and hyperosmolality may occur with prolonged use. Mannitol is normally administered at a dose of 0.25 to 1.0 g kg^{-1} as a 20% gravity-driven infusion. Large boluses of more concentrated mannitol may lead to hyperosmolarity-induced cerebral vasodilatation and further increases in ICP (Cottrell, Robustelli and Post, 1977).

Loop diuretics, such as frusemide (furosemide) (1 mg kg^{-1} i.v.), reduce ICP by causing brain dehydration through diuresis, and by decreasing CSF production (Wilkinson, Wepsic and Austen, 1971). Although the onset of action of frusemide is slower than that of mannitol (about 30 to 45 minutes), this agent has the advantage of decreasing ICP without increasing blood osmolality or intravascular volume. This would be desirable in patients with congestive heart failure. Combined therapy employing both frusemide and mannitol may be used in extreme circumstances to rapidly decrease ICP, but risks potentially dangerous electrolyte and intravascular volume depletion.

Corticosteroids are commonly used to treat cerebral oedema. Postulated mechanisms of action include repair of the blood–brain barrier, prevention of deleterious lysosomal activity, enhancement of cerebral electrolyte transport, improvement in cerebral metabolism and promotion of electrolyte and water excretion (Bouzarth and Shenkin, 1974). The clinical efficacy of corticosteroids for treating cerebral oedema is as yet unproven, but appears to be of benefit in reducing oedema secondary to brain tumours and hydrocephalus. Corticosteroids appear to have a protective effect if given before damage occurs. These agents are commonly recommended before intracranial surgery to reduce postoperative inflammation and oedema formation (Franklin, 1984).

Hyperventilation to decrease $Paco_2$ is also efficacious in reducing ICP, but should be applied in such a way as to minimize increases in mean intrathoracic pressure (Shapiro, 1986b). Excessive inflation pressure or prolonged inspiratory time may compound the situation by causing unnecessary increases in central venous pressure thereby increasing ICP. This can be managed, to some extent, by repositioning the patient so that the patient's head is above the chest level and by avoiding extreme flexion or twisting of the neck.

Systemic blood pressure control using hypotensive agents, such as sodium nitroprusside, and use of cerebral vasoconstrictors, such as the barbiturates, are treatments reserved for more extreme cases of intracranial hypertension. Increased ICP resulting from hydrocephalus may be alleviated using acetazolamide to reduce the rate of CSF production, by the use of osmotic agents (such as mannitol) and by surgical CSF diversion (Shapiro, 1986b). Intracranial masses should be removed surgically where possible.

ANAESTHESIA AND SEIZURES

Pathophysiology of seizures

A seizure has been defined as a stereotypic alteration in behaviour resulting from the paroxysmal discharge of a group of abnormal neurons in the brain (Oliver & Lorenz, 1987). Such abnormal behaviour may include loss of consciousness, change in muscle tone or movement, alteration in sensory perception (e.g. hallucinations), alteration in autonomic control, other abnormal moods, or a combination of these behaviours. Epilepsy is a syndrome of recurring seizures (Oliver and Lorenz, 1987).

Seizures are commonly classified based on clinical presentation. Focal (or partial) seizures result in clinical signs compatible with a localized area of neuronal dysfunction such as marked changes in behaviour, aggression or apparent hallucination. Generalized seizures are commonly paroxysmal and associated with loss of consciousness. Most generalized seizures observed in small animals present as violent muscular activity (grand mal seizures). Less commonly, sudden loss of consciousness may be all that is observed (petit mal seizures).

Seizures are not a disease, rather they are the clinical manifestation of disorders of neuronal dysfunction (Bunch, 1986). They may reflect a systemic illness which manifests as CNS dysfunction or may result directly from intracranial disease. Although the biochemical mechanisms involved in the genesis of seizures are, as yet, not clearly understood, the fundamental event may be a disturbance of CNS excitability resulting in a focus of excessive neuronal discharge (Stoelting, Dierdorf and McCammon, 1988). This area may remain localized if surrounded by neurons which are hyperpolarized. If the stimulus is large enough, surrounding neurons are recruited resulting in massive synchronous discharges and generalized seizures. Table 2 lists some common causes of seizures in small animals.

The level of stimulation required to initiate a seizure is known as the seizure threshold. Drugs, such as acepromazine, decrease the seizure threshold and therefore increase an animal's susceptibility to seizure. Agents which elevate the seizure threshold, such as phenobarbitone, are commonly used in the medical management of seizure disorders.

Grand mal seizures can have significant sequelae for the anaesthetist. While the seizure persists, metabolic activity and oxygen consumption is increased both systemically and within the central nervous system. This, coupled with airway obstruction and ineffective chest wall movements, result in respiratory and metabolic acidosis and hypoxaemia. Hyperthermia also results from excessive muscular activity. As a result of these changes, intracranial pressure will be increased and may become clinically significant in animals with intracranial pathology. If the seizure process is not terminated, such as in the case of status epilepticus, arterial hypotension and death may follow. Permanent neuronal degeneration has resulted from frequent, prolonged seizures (Shapiro, 1986a).

Table 2.   Causes of seizures

Classification	Examples
Iatrogenic	Drugs (myelographic contrast agents, ketamine, methohexitone)
Congenital	Hydrocephalus
Degenerative	Storage diseases
Infectious	Canine distemper, feline infectious peritonitis, toxoplasmosis, cryptococcosis
Metabolic	Hypocalacaemia, hypoglycaemia, uraemia
Neoplastic	Intracranial tumour
Nutritional	Thiamine deficiency
Toxic	Heavy metals, strychnine
Unknown	Idiopathic epilepsy

Anaesthesia and the seizure prone patient

Selection of anaesthetic agents for the seizure prone patient must consider the impact of anticonvulsant therapy on organ function (Stoelting, Dierdorf and McCammon, 1988). Table 3 lists commonly used anticonvulsant agents and their known adverse side effects. Many of these agents induce CNS depression particularly when used at the high end of the therapeutic dose range. Because of this, sedative anaesthetic agents will have exaggerated effects when administered at the usual dosages. In addition, many anticonvulsant agents stimulate hepatic metabolic activity and may increase the rate of metabolism and decrease the duration of effect of many anaesthetic agents. An adverse sequela to this is that the hepatotoxic and/or nephrotoxic potential of some agents, such as methoxyflurane, may be enhanced. For these reasons, patients on anticonvulsant therapy should receive reduced dosages of sedative agents. The duration of action of these drugs is likely to be shorter than expected.

Anaesthetic premedicants should be selected for direct anticonvulsant effects, or at least, lack of seizurogenic potential. In this light, a benzodiazepine such as diazepam (0.1–0.4 mg kg^{-1} i.m.) or midazolam (0.1–0.4 mg kg^{-1} i.m.) may be included in the preanaesthetic regimen. It is generally inadvisable to use these drugs alone because of the risk of inducing paradoxical excitement. However, they may be used to supplement the sedative effects of opioid agents such as butorphanol (0.1–0.2 mg kg^{-1} i.m.) or pethidine

Table 3. Commonly used anticonvulsant agents

Agent	Use	Dose	Other effects
Diazepam	Status epilepticus	0.2–0.5 mg kg^{-1} i.v. to effect	
Pentobarbitone	Status epilepticus	10–15 mg kg^{-1} i.v. to effect	Produces profound sedation or anaesthesia. Irritant if injected perivascularly
Phenobarbitone	Status epilepticus Generalized grand mal and partial seizures	10 mg kg^{-1} i.v. 0.5–5 mg kg^{-1} by mouth twice a day	Increases metabolism of other drugs. Elevates serum liver enzyme activity. Polydipsia, polyuria, polyphagia
Primidone	Generalized grand mal and partial seizures	5–15 mg kg^{-1} by mouth three times a day (dogs only)	Metabolized to phenobarbitone. Elevates serum liver enzyme activity. Reports of liver cirrhosis/ necrosis. Sedative effects enhanced by chloramphenicol, cortisol, some opioid agents, phenothiazines, phenylbutazone and digitalis
Phenytoin	Generalized grand mal and partial seizures (not considered to be very effective in small animals)	30–50 mg kg^{-1} by mouth three times a day (dogs only)	Liver toxicity. Sedative effects enhanced by chloramphenicol. Megaloblastic anaemia caused by folate deficiency

(meperidine) (3–5 mg kg^{-1} i.m.). When used at premedicant dosages, most opioid agents will not promote seizure activity (Shapiro, 1986a). At higher dosages, morphine, pethidine, pentazocine and fentanyl have been reported to induce seizures (Shapiro, 1986a). The phenothiazines and cyclohexamines, such as ketamine and tiletamine, have been implicated as agents which promote seizure activity and should be omitted from the anaesthetic protocol for patients prone to seizure (Booth, 1982; Wright, 1982).

Intravenous induction with a thiobarbiturate is acceptable in most situations. The ultrashort- and short-acting barbiurates are not anticonvulsants, *per se*, but they control seizures by virtue of their anaesthetic activity. Methohexitone, an oxybarbiturate, may induce myoclonus and seizures if the patient's consciousness is not adequately depressed by sedative premedication (Ford, Morrell and Whisler, 1982; Wauquier *et al.*, 1978). This drug is probably best avoided in seizure prone patients. Ketamine is contraindicated as it has been shown to initiate seizures in epileptic as well as normal patients (Ferrer-Allado, Brechner and Dymond, 1973). Saffan appears to be safe for induction of seizure prone cats.

Most of the inhaled anaesthetics have been reported to produce seizures although the occurrence of postanaesthetic seizures appears to be quite rare (Stoelting, Dierdorf and McCammon, 1988). Of all the agents, enflurane is associated with the highest incidence of seizure activity in dogs and cats, especially if administered at inspired concentrations greater than 1.5 MAC or if used in patients that are hypercapnic or hypocapnic (Michenfelder and Cucchiaria, 1974; Clark and Rosner, 1973). Isoflurane appears to be the inhalational agent of choice for use in the seizure prone patient because of a low incidence of seizures in clinical patients and because this agent causes minimal changes in cerebral haemodynamics (Stoelting, Dierdorf and McCammon, 1988).

Management of the seizuring patient

Repeated generalized seizures in a short period of time without recovery comprise status epilepticus (Bunch, 1986). Animals in status epilepticus should be treated without delay to minimize immediate and long-term detrimental effects associated with hypoxic neuronal damage, acidosis and hyperthermia. Initial therapy should include administration of diazepam (0.1–0.4 mg kg^{-1} i.v.) in incremental doses until the animal responds. If diazepam is ineffective (usually after three doses), then phenobarbitone (10 mg kg^{-1} i.v.) should be given. If neither is effective, then pentobarbitone (10–15 mg kg^{-1} i.v.) should be administered slowly to effect. Pentobarbitone should be administered cautiously since both diazepam and phenobarbitone will potentiate its effect. When the animal is sufficiently relaxed, a patent airway should be ensured by endotracheal intubation, and adequate oxygenation and ventilation provided. Body temperature, blood pressure, and arterial blood gas tensions should be assessed and corrected if found to be abnormal. The initiating cause of the seizures should be identified, where possible, and treated.

REFERENCES

Booth, N. H. (1982). In *Veterinary Pharmacology and Therapeutics*, 5th edn, eds. N. H. Booth and L. E. McDonald, p. 331. Ames, Iowa: Iowa State University Press.

Bouzarth, W. F. and Shenkin, H. A. (1974). *Journal of Trauma* 14, 134.

Bunch, S. E. (1986). In *Current Veterinary Therapy IX, Small Animal Practice*, ed. R. W. Kirk, p. 836. Philadelphia: W. B. Saunders Co.

Campkin, T. V. and Turner, J. M. (1980). In Neurosurgical Anaesthesia and Intensive Care, p. 129. Boston: Butterworth.

Clark, D. L. and Rosner, B. S. (1973). *Anesthesiology* 38, 564.

Cottrell, J. E., Robustelli, A. and Post, K. (1977). *Anesthesiology* 47, 28.

Ferrer-Allado, T., Brechner, V. L. and Dymond, A. (1973). *Anesthesiology* 38, 333.

Fitch, W., Burke, J. and McDowall, D. G. (1969). *British Journal of Anaesthesia* 41, 564.

Ford, E. W., Morrell, F. and Whisler, W. W. (1982). *Anesthesia and Analgesia* 61, 997.

Franklin, R. T. (1984). *The Compendium on Continuing Education for the Practicing Veterinarian* 6, 442.

Hougaard, K., Hansen, A. and Brodersen, P. (1974). *Anesthesiology* 41, 562.

Kuschinsky, W. and Wahl, M. (1978). *Physiology Review* 58, 565.

LeCouteur, R. A. and Turrel, J. M. (1986). In *Current Veterinary Therapy IX, Small Animal Practice*, ed. R. W. Kirk, p. 820. Philadelphia: W. B. Saunders Co.

Maekawa, T., Sakabe, T. and Takeshita, H. (1974). *Anesthesiology* 41, 389.

McPherson, R. W. and Traystman, R. J. (1984). *Anesthesiology* 60, 180.

Michenfelder, J. D. and Cucchiaria, R. F. (1974). *Anesthesiology* 40, 575.

Misfeldt, B. B., Jorgensen, P. B. and Spotoft, H. (1976). *British Journal of Anaesthesia* 48, 963.

Oliver, J. E. and Lorenz, M. D. (1987). In *Handbook of Veterinary Neurologic Diagnosis*, eds. J. E. Oliver and M. D. Lorenz, p. 289. Philadelphia: W. B. Saunders.

Pickerodt, V. W. A., McDowall, D. G., Coroneos, N. J. and Keany, N. P. (1972). *British Journal of Anaesthesia* 44, 751.

Pierce, E. C., Lambertsen, C. J. and Deutsch, S. (1962). *Journal of Clinical Investigation* 41, 1664.

Sakabe, T., Kuramoto, T. and Kumagae, S. (1976). *Anesthesiology* 48, 195.

Shapiro, H. M. (1986a). In *Anesthesia*, 2nd edn, ed. R. D. Miller, p. 1249. New York: Churchill Livingstone.

Shapiro, H. M. (1986b). In *Anesthesia*, 2nd edn, ed. R. D. Miller, p. 1563. New York: Churchill Livingstone.

Siesjo, B. K. (1984). *Journal of Neurosurgery* **60**, 883.

Stoelting, R. K., Dierdorf, S. F. and McCammon, R. L. (1988). In *Anesthesia and Co-Existing Disease*, 2nd edn, p. 263. New York: Churchill Livingstone.

Tabbador, K. (1986). In *Anesthesia and Neurosurgery*, 2nd edn, eds. J. E. Cottrell and H. Turndorf, p. 43. St Louis: The C. V. Mosby Co.

Takeshita, H., Michenfelder, J. D. and Theye, R. A. (1972). *Anesthesiology* **37**, 605.

Vinall, P. E. and Simeone, F. A. (1981). *Stroke* **12**, 640.

Wauquier, A., Vanden Broeck, W. A., Verheyer, J. L. and Janssen, P. A. (1978). *European Journal of Pharmacology* **47**, 367.

Wilkinson, H. A., Wepsic, J. G. and Austen, G. (1971). *Journal of Neurosurgery* **34**, 203.

Wright, M. (1982). *Journal of the American Medical Association* **180**, 1462.

11

Anaesthesia for patients with central nervous system disease: specific disease situations and their management

With the advent of modern neurodiagnostic techniques, such as computed tomography and magnetic resonance imaging, anaesthesia is more commonly required for the diagnostic and surgical management of small animal patients with neurological impairment. Perhaps in no other area of veterinary anaesthesia is the selection and application of anaesthetic agents as likely to influence outcome as it does in these patients.

This chapter describes comprehensive anaesthetic management strategies for small animal patients with specific types of neurological disease. The management of the neurological patient for a number of diagnostic procedures is also discussed.

INTRACRANIAL TUMOURS

Neoplasia of the central nervous system is no longer considered uncommon in domestic animals (Braund, 1987). Although the exact occurrence of intracranial tumours in animals is unknown, the incidence rate has been estimated at 14.5 cases per 100 000 population for dogs and 3.5 cases per 100 000 population for cats, which is comparable to estimates for man (LeCouteur and Turrel, 1986; Stoelting, Dierdorf and McCammon, 1988).

Older brachycephalic dogs, especially of the Boxer, English Bulldog and Boston Terrier breeds, have the highest incidence of brain tumours amongst the domestic animals (Fankhauser, Luginbuhl and McGrath, 1974; Hayes and Schiefer, 1969). The most common primary brain tumours in dogs are meningiomas, gliomas and undifferentiated sarcomas, while meningiomas are the most commonly reported primary brain tumours in the cat (Hayes and

Schiefer, 1969; Nafe, 1979). A multiplicity of secondary tumours is also found.

Clinical signs are dependent on the location and rate of growth of the neoplasm. Localized (or focal) signs associated with the direct compressive or irritative effects of the tumour are seen most frequently and may include hemiparesis, circling, hemisensory abnormalities and focal or generalized seizures. Generalized (or non-focal) signs often result from secondary effects of the tumour, such as increased intracranial pressure (ICP), and may include depressed mentation, behavioural changes, head pressing, pacing and papilloedema (LeCouteur and Turrel, 1986).

The presence and approximate location of an intracranial tumour may be determined by history, physical and neurological examination. Definitive diagnosis of a tumour usually requires additional diagnostic aids such as cerebrospinal fluid (CSF) analysis, electroencephalography (EEG), plain and contrast radiography and computed tomography (CT). Computed tomography, although limited to veterinary teaching institutions and human hospitals that will scan animals, provides one of the most accurate methods for spatial localization of a brain tumour (LeCouteur and Turrel, 1986).

Treatment of intracranial neoplasia may involve complete eradication of the tumour or at least palliative reduction in tumour mass by either surgery, radiation therapy, chemotherapy, immunotherapy, or a combination of these methods (LeCouteur and Turrel, 1986; Turrel, Fike and LeCouteur, 1984). With the increase in availabiliy of spatial imaging modalities (such as CT) and the development of advanced neurosurgical and neuroanaesthetic techniques, surgery is more frequently used for the excision of accessible tumours (such as meningiomas) or at least for biopsy and/or debulking prior to definitive therapy (Braund, 1987).

Anaesthetic management

Optimal management of anaesthesia for patients with brain tumours necessitates a thorough understanding of the normal cerebral circulation, the changes in circulatory response that may occur with an intracranial mass and of the interactions of anaestheic agents and techniques with the disturbed circulation (Stoelting, Dierdorf and McCammon, 1988).

Expansion of an intracranial neoplasm will result in a decrease in intracranial compliance (a shift to the right along the cerebral pressure–volume compliance curve). Small increases in intracranial volume, which may occur during anaesthesia, can result in large increases in intracranial pressure, thereby jeopardizing adequate cerebral circulation. In addition, regional cerebral blood flow is likely to be abnormal in animals with brain tumours. The tissue within and immediately surrounding the tumour is likely to contain blood vessels which have lost vasomotor control and are maximally dilated from the low pH of metabolites generated by the tumour. This results in so-called 'luxury perfusion' (Lassen, 1966). If the $Paco_2$ is allowed to increase (by hypoventilation) blood flow will be shunted away from these tissues resulting in an intracerebral steal syndrome which may compromise the circulation to the tumour and surrounding tissues. Conversely, if the $Paco_2$ decreases (by hyperventilation) blood flow will be redirected towards the tumour. This response has been termed the inverse steal or 'Robin Hood' phenomenon (Samuels, 1986). The clinical significance of these phenomena is unknown. However the prudent approach would be to avoid situations which promote hypoventilation in the awake animal and to induce mild hypocapnia ($Paco_2$ 25 to 30 mmHg) by mechanical ventilation in the anaesthetized patient.

Preanaesthetic evaluation of the patient with a brain tumour centres around detection of signs of intracranial hypertension. These may include alterations in level of consciousness, pupillary dilatation, decreased pupillary light reflex, papilloedema, bradycardia, hypertension and disturbances in respiration. Computed tomography may provide evidence of a midline shift of the brain which also suggests the presence of increased intracranial pressure. Definitive measurement of CSF pressure may have been performed if a cisternal tap was included as part of the diagnostic work-up. Normal CSF pressure is between 6 and 17 cmH_2O. Pressure readings in animals with brain tumours may be as high as 30 cmH_2O (Indrieri and Simpson, 1985).

Animals with evidence of intracranial hypertension should be treated with corticosteroids (dexamethasone or methylprednisolone) before surgery. Routine use of corticosteroids before and after surgery has been shown to significantly reduce mortality rates in human patients undergoing the removal of brain tumours (Stoelting, Dierdorf and McCammon, 1988). Hyperosmotic agents (such as mannitol at 1 g kg^{-1} slow i.v.) may be indicated if neurological signs do not abate before surgery with corticosteroids alone. It should be remembered that the effects of the hyperosmotic drugs are relatively transient and may be contraindicated in patients with an incomplete blood-brain barrier. Furthermore, it has been suggested that frusemide (furosemide) (1 mg kg^{-1} i.v.) may be more effective at controlling intraoperative increases in intracranial pressure than mannitol, particularly if the blood-brain barrier is altered (Cottrell *et al.*, 1977).

Occasionally, patients may present with evidence of pituitary involvement which manifests as abnormalities of endocrine production such as hypothyroidism, secondary adrenal failure or diabetes insipidus. These abnormalities should be corrected as far as possible before surgery. The anaesthetic management of animals with endocrine disease has been discussed previously (Court et al., 1988).

Patients with intracranial tumours may present with a history of seizures requiring therapy. Ideally, seizures should be controlled prior to anaesthesia. Phenobarbitone (1–2 mg kg^{-1} orally every 12 hours) appears to be the drug of choice (LeCouteur and Turrel, 1986).

Anaesthetic premedication is beneficial in patients with brain tumours to alleviate anxiety and smooth induction and recovery. Stress or excitement should be avoided because sympathetic activation may elevate intracranial pressure. Agents which depress ventilation should also be avoided. It should be remembered that animals with intracranial pathology may be extremely sensitive to central nervous system depressant drugs. In this regard, a small dose of an opioid agent such as pethidine (1–3 mg kg^{-1} i.m.) or butorphanol (0.1–0.2 mg kg^{-1} i.m.) may be all that is required. For the seizure-prone patient, a benzodiazepine such as diazepam (0.1–0.2 mg kg^{-1} i.m.) or midazolam (0.1–0.2 mg kg^{-1} i.m.) may be added or substituted. Phenothiazine derivatives should be avoided because of the propensity for hypotension which may compromise cerebral blood flow and because of increased risk of seizures. Lethargic, obtunded patients will not require sedative premedication. Antcholinergic agents such as glycopyrronium (glycopyrrolate) (0.01 mg kg^{-1} i.m.) should be administered in combination with any opioid agent and may be required to treat animals with pre-existent bradydysrhythmias.

All animals should be preoxygenated by face mask before induction of anaesthesia to reduce the likelihood of cerebral hypoxia at intubation. Induction of anaesthesia should be rapid and smooth in order to minimize effects on cerebral blood flow. Intubation of the trachea should be accomplished rapidly without stimulating a cough or gagging response. In cats, the larynx should be sprayed with a topical lignocaine solution to suppress laryngeal spasm, coughing or gagging reflexes during intubation. In man, intravenous lignocaine has been shown to be more efficacious than topical administration for preventing increases in ICP during intubation (Hamill, Bedford and Weaver 1981). However, intravenous lignocaine was not shown to be effective in suppressing these protective responses in cats (Dyson, 1988). In most instances, intravenous induction with a thiobarbiturate, such as thiopentone (8–10 mg kg^{-1} to effect) or thiamylal (8–10 mg kg^{-1} to effect), is satisfactory. Thiobarbiturates have the advantage of being potent cerebral vasoconstrictors. They also decrease cerebral metabolic rate while increasing the cerebral perfusion to metabolism ratio. Ketamine should be avoided because it promotes cerebral vasodilatation and increases CSF pressure. This response is also exaggerated in patients with intracranial pathology (Bennett, Madsen and Jordan, 1973).

Immediately following endotracheal intubation, the animal should be mechanically ventilated using a respiratory rate and tidal volume calculated to maintain the $Paco_2$ between 25 and 30 mmHg (approximately 10 breaths min^{-1} respiratory rate and 20–30 ml kg^{-1} tidal volume). Where possible, $Paco_2$ should be substantiated by arterial blood gas measurement. Hypocapnia will decrease cerebral blood flow and CSF pressure.

Anaesthesia is best maintained using minimal doses of volatile inhalational agents. All of the volatile anaesthetic agents cause dose-dependent cerebral vasodilatation which can be obtunded by hypocapnia. Isoflurane appears to be the inhalational agent of choice as it has minimal effects on CBF and ICP (Stoelting, Dierdorf and McCammon, 1988). Halothane may be used if hyperventilation of the patient is initiated before introduction of the agent into the inhaled mixture. Nitrous oxide is not recommended in animals undergoing craniotomy because of the possibility of exacerbation of venous air embolism from the cut edge of the skull (Stoelting, Dierdorf and McCammon, 1988).

The use of skeletal muscle relaxants is beneficial in patients with increased ICP, to facilitate mechanical ventilation of the lungs, to prevent reflex movements of the animal in response to surgery, and to minimize the concentration (and adverse physiological effects) of the inhalational anaesthetic agent. Vecuronium (0.05–0.1 mg kg^{-1} i.v.) and atracurium (0.2–0.4 mg kg^{-1} i.v.) appear to be the relaxants of choice because they have been shown to have minimal effects on intracranial pressure in patients with brain tumours (Rosa, Orfei and Sanfilippo, 1986; Rosa, Sanfilippo and Vilardi, 1986). Agents which provoke histamine release, such as *d*-tubocurarine or high doses of atracurium, should be avoided since histamine is a potent cerebral vasodilator (Stoelting, Dierdorf and McCammon, 1988). It should be remembered that there may be increased resistance to neuromuscular blockade in limbs which are paretic as a result of the brain tumour. Therefore, when using a nerve stimulator to monitor the degree of muscle paralysis, a non-paretic limb should be used or else relative overdose of the relaxant may ensue (Moorthy and Hilgenberg, 1980).

Selection of the type and rate of administration of intravenous fluids is critical in these patients. Solutions containing dextrose, in particular 5% dextrose in water, should be avoided because of the tendency for these to increase brain water content, promote cerebral oedema formation and lead to poorer neurological outcome. Hyperosmotic soluions such as dextran 70 have been recommended to reduce brain water content (Stoelting, Dierdorf and McCammon, 1988). If balanced electrolyte solutions, such as lactated Ringer's solution, are used, the rate of fluid administration should not exceed 1–3 ml kg^{-1} h^{-1}. Intraoperative blood losses should be replaced by either whole blood or colloid solutions (such as dextran 70).

Anaesthetic depth should be monitored closely, especially in the paralysed patient. Blood pressure should be maintained within normal limits. Hypertension (>100 mmHg mean arterial pressure) may indicate inadequate anaesthetic depth and result in deleterious increases in CSF pressure, while hypotension (<60mmHg mean) may result in cerebral ischaemia. The electrocardiogram should be monitored to detect cardiac dysrhythmias related to intracranial hypertension or surgical manipulation. Abnormalities may range from acute sinus bradycardia to ventricular ectopic beats or tachycardia.

Animals undergoing craniotomy are normally positioned in sternal recumbency. Slight elevation of the head (10 to 15 degrees) will facilitate venous drainage. Excessive elevation of the head should be avoided since this may predispose to venous air embolism. The cut edge of the skull is a common site for entry of air into veins held open by bone (Stoelting, Dierdorf and McCammon, 1988). Following venous air embolism, death may occur from either obstruction of right ventricular ejection or of coronary arterial flow. Neurological damage will follow air embolism to the brain. Signs of air embolism include paroxysmal inspiratory effects by the patient ('gasps'), hypotension, tachycardia, cardiac dysrhyhmias and cyanosis. A characteristic 'mill-wheel' murmur may be auscultated (Gilroy and Anson, 1987; Michenfelder, 1983). These are usually late signs of catastrophic air embolism. More sensitive indicators of air embolism include measurement of end-tidal carbon dioxide concentration (capnography) and use of a right heart Doppler transducer (Stoelting, Dierdorf and McCammon, 1988). Specific treatment involves identification and occlusion of the site of air entry by irrigation of the operative site and application of an occlusive material to the bone edges (Stoelting, Dierdorf and McCammon, 1988). Air may be aspirated from the right heart if a central venous line has been previously placed. Nitrous oxide, if used, should be immediately discontinued. Positive end-expiratory pressure may help by increasing venous pressure. Secondary effects of air embolism such as hypotension and cardiac dysrhythmias should be treated symptomatically.

Anaesthetic recovery should be as smooth as possible in order to avoid intracranial pressure increases associated with excitement or coughing. This may be facilitated by administration of supplemental doses of a mild sedative and analgesic agent, such as butorphanol (0.05 mg kg^{-1} i.v.), at the time of extubation. Early extubation, before a coughing reflex has returned, is also indicated provided an adequate airway can be maintained by the patient. The neurological status of these patents should be monitored closely during the postoperative period to facilitate early detection of complications such as intracranial haemorrhage, oedema or infarction.

HEAD INJURY

Traumatic injuries to the head are commonly encountered in small animal patients (Fenner, 1986). In one study, it was found that approximately 20% of traumatic injuries in dogs and 35% in cats involved the head (Kolata, Kraut and Johnston, 1974). Head injuries may involve damage to the central nervous system (brain), peripheral nervous system (cranial nerves), or both. Cranial nerve injuries are usually permanent but rarely life-threatening. On the other hand, injuries to the brain are often life-threatening but are likely to result in fewer long-term complications (Fenner, 1986).

Mortality in patients with head trauma may result from either the primary head injury, secondary effects of the head injury or from non-neural traumatic injury. Primary head injury results from the biomechanical effect of the forces applied to the skull at the time of traumatic insult and is manifested within milliseconds of the insult (Bruce, 1986). Generally, patients that survive long enough to reach a veterinary hospital do not die from the primary insult. Secondary neuronal damage in these patients commences immediately following the primary insult. A vicious circle is initiated by oedema formation, intracranial haemorrhage and possibly by direct effects on the cardiorespiratory control centres. These may result in hypoventilation, hypoxia, hypertension and increased intracranial pressure all of which further compromise localized and global neuronal blood supply and oxygenation. Non-neural injuries, particularly those involving the cardiorespiratory system, may further complicate secondary neuronal damage, or if severe enough may directly cause the death of the animal.

Preliminary evaluation and treatment of these patients involves detection and correction of life-threatening non-neural injuries. These may include pneumothorax, major internal or external haemorrhage and traumatic cardiac dysrhythmias. Shock invariably accompanies major corporeal insults and will further complicate intracranial damage. Colloid solutions such as dextran 70 (10–20 ml kg^{-1} i.v.) or whole blood (in the case of haemorrhagic shock) should be used instead of large volumes of crystalloid to treat shock in these animals so as not to aggravate intracranial swelling.

Following emergency stabilization of the patient, a thorough physical and neurological examination should be performed to detect and evaluate the suspected head injury. In particular, the skull should be palpated for fractures, and the animal's level of consciousness, pupil size and symmetry, and presence or absence of physiological nystagmus should be noted (Fenner, 1986). These latter tests help differentiate between cerebral and brain stem injury. Brain stem injury holds a poorer prognosis. Other diagnostic tests which may be used to define the injury include skull radiography and CT scan.

Medical therapy of these animals may involve administration of corticosteroids, oxygen, and general supportive care (Fenner, 1986). Patients that seizure require treatment with either diazepam or phenobarbitone. Mannitol should only be used as a last resort to decrease intracranial pressure in these animals, because of the likelihood of an incomplete blood–brain barrier. Frusemide (furosemide) may be beneficial in this situation. Surgery may be required for treatment of depressed skull fractures and epidural or subdural haemotomas. In addition, animals may require anaesthesia for immobilization during radiography and CT scan.

Anaesthetic management

Common pathophysiological changes induced by acute head injury which may impact on anaesthesia include hypoventilation, hypoxaemia, hypertension, tachycardia, cardiac dysrrhythmias and intracranial hypertension (Matjasko, 1986; Miner and Allen, 1984). Less common but important sequelae include neurogenic pulmonary oedema, disseminated intravascular coagulation, fibrinolysis syndrome and a multiplicity of endocrine abnormalities (Matjasko, 1986). Anaesthetic management of these patients should be directed at improving arterial oxygenation and cardiopulmonary function and optimizing intracranial dynamics.

Preanaesthetic assessment of these animals should include cardiopulmonary evaluation and estimation of the degree of intracranial hypertension by physical and neurological examination. Arterial blood gas analysis, evaluation of the electrocardiogram (ECG) and arterial blood pressure measurement are useful diagnostic aids. Hypoxaemic animals (Pao_2 <80 mmHg) will require perioperative oxygen supplementation, while hypercapnic patients ($Paco_2$ >45 mmHg) should be mechanically ventilated. Arterial hypertension and tachycardia has been reported to occur in more than 30% of severely head injured human patients (Brown, Mohr and Carey, 1967). Because of the deleterious effects of hypertension on intracranial pressure, the use of β-adrenergic antagonists, such as propranolol, has been advocated in these patients. Cardiac dysrhythmias usually relate to hypoxaemia or autonomic system activation and therefore often respond to oxygen therapy or antidysrhythmic drugs. The presence of intracranial hypertension is a prognostic indicator associated with a poor outcome (Frost, 1986). Preoperative therapy may involve administration of corticosteroids such as dexamethasone (2–4 mg kg⁻¹ i.v.) and diuretics such as frusemide (1 mg kg⁻¹ i.v.). Mechanical hyperventilation is indicated in unresponsive, hypercapnic patients.

Sedative premedication is rarely indicated since these patients are usually neurologically obtunded and it is important to avoid further cardiorespiratory depression. Small doses of opioid agents, such as butorphanol (0.1–0.2 mg kg⁻¹ i.m.) or pethidine (3–5 mg kg⁻¹ i.m.), may be beneficial in painful patients to reduce perioperative stress.

Anaesthetic induction should be accomplished as expeditiously and atraumatically as possible using incremental doses of an ultrashort-acting barbiturate, such as thiamylal or thiopentone (8–10 mg kg⁻¹ i.v.). The animal should be intubated with a snug-fitting endotracheal tube and hyperventilation should be initiated in order to achieve a $Paco_2$ of 25 to 30 mmHg. Anaesthesia is best maintained with minimal levels of isoflurane. Nitrous oxide should be avoided because of the risk of increasing the size of a trapped air mass. The use of a skeletal muscle relaxant such as vecuronium or atracurium is advocated to minimize inhalant anaesthetic dose. Intravenous fluid replacement should be with balanced electrolyte solutions.

Important aspects regarding monitoring these patients include frequent assessment of anaesthetic depth, continuous monitoring of the ECG and arterial pressure measurement. It is particularly important to maintain normal blood pressure, and therefore cerebral perfusion, in these animals. Hypertension related to inadequate anaesthetic depth should be treated by increasing the delivered inhalant anaesthetic concentration or, more ideally, by administering supplemental intravenous doses of an opioid agent. Hypotension may be treated effectively by administering colloid solutions such as dextran 70 (10–20 ml kg⁻¹ i.v.).

Recovery from anaesthesia should be as smooth as possible. Extubation is accomplished once the animal is able to maintain an airway.

DECOMPRESSIVE SPINAL SURGERY

Surgical diseases affecting spinal cord function include interverte-bral disc disease, discospondylitis, fractures and luxations of the spinal column, cervical malformation and malarticulation, and neoplasia of the cord or surrounding tissues (Walker and Betts, 1985; Walker *et al.*, 1985).

Of these conditions, protrusion or extrusion of the intervertebral discs into the spinal canal occurs most frequently. Chondrodystro-phoid breeds such as the Dachshund, Pekingese and Beagle are particularly susceptible. Lesions most often involve the thoraco-lumbar spine with the T12–T13 interspace being the most common site of disc rupture. Approximately 25% of cases involve the cervical spine with C2–C3 being the most common site for disc rupture to occur. Clinical signs observed commonly include hyper-pathia and neurological dysfunction ranging from mild paresis to paralysis of affected limbs. Diagnosis is based on history, neuro-logical examination, and plain and contrast radiography of the spinal column. Treatment initially involves confinement of the animal and judicious use of anti-inflammatory drugs. Animals that fail to respond to medical therapy and continue to degenerate usually require surgery to remove extruded disc material and decompress the spinal cord (Walker and Betts, 1985).

Discospondylitis results from either haematogenous or foreign body spread of infections to the intervertebral disc. Neurological deficits occur primarily because of spinal cord compression by new bone and fibrous connective tissue growth. Occasionally, deficits may be caused by vertebral subluxation resulting from instability, or by extension of the infection to the spinal cord and meninges. Diagnosis is based on clinical signs and radiographic findings. Treatment of patients with little or no neurological deficit usually involves parenteral antibiotic therapy. Animals with pronounced neurological signs and myelographic evidence of cord compression require decompressive surgery via hemilaminectomy (Walker *et al.*, 1985).

Fractures and luxations of the spinal column commonly result from traumatic injury. Surgery may be required for decompression of the spinal cord by reduction and stabilization of the lesion or by laminectomy.

Cervical malformation and malarticulation is a disease of large breeds of dog, such as the Great Dane and Doberman Pinscher, which is characterized by a slowly progressive ascending tetrapa-resis and ataxia (Walker *et al.*, 1985). Definitive diagnosis is based on cervical radiographs and myelography. Conservative treatment involves restriction of activities and use of anti-inflammatory drugs. Surgical treatment may be used to decompress the spinal cord and stabilize involved vertebral segments.

Spinal tumours are most commonly extradural in location (50% of cases) and are generally primary vertebral tumours including osteosarcomas, fibrosarcomas and chondrosarcomas (Kornegay, 1985). These tumours grow rapidly resulting in an acute and progressive paresis. Meningiomas and neurofibromas are the most common intradural, extramedullary tumours (20% of cases). Initially they may only compress a single nerve root resulting in monoparesis, but subsequently they often compress the spinal cord resulting in paraparesis or tetraparesis. Intradural intramedullary tumours (30% of cases) are either primary neural or metastatic in origin. Their course varies from acute to insidious. Diagnosis of spinal tumours is based on history, plain film radiography, myelography and CT (if available). Surgery is often required for definitive diagnosis and treatment, provided the tumour is amenable to excision.

Anaesthetic management

Spinal cord blood flow appears to respond to fluctuations in arterial pressure and $Paco_2$ in a way analogous to cerebral blood flow regulation (Kornegay, 1985). In one study, spinal cord perfusion was reduced by 50% when mean arterial pressure decreased to 50 mmHg. Spinal cord perfusion ceased when mean arterial pressure reached 30 mmHg. Trauma to the spinal cord has been shown to abolish both chemical regulation and pressure autoregulation of spinal cord blood flow (Kobrine, Doyle and Martins, 1975). Anaesthetic management of these patients should therefore be designed to optimize both cardiovascular and respiratory function in an attempt to minimize ischaemic damage to the spinal cord.

Corticosteroid therapy appears to be beneficial in reducing the degree of spinal cord damage, especially if initiated immediately following the injury, or prior to surgery in the case of chronic lesions (Rucker, Lumb and Scott, 1981). Mannitol has also been used to reduce cord oedema, although the beneficial effects may be short-lived. Other forms of treatment, which are as yet unproven or experimental, include the use of localized hypothermia, hyperbaric oxygenation, catecholamine antagonists, dimethyl sulphoxide (DMSO) and opioid antagonists such as naloxone and thyrotropin releasing hormone (Albin, White and Acosta-Rua, 1968; Faden, Jacobs and Holaday, 1981; Faden *et al.*, 1981; Hartzog, Fischer and Snow, 1971; Kajihara, Kawanaga and de la Torre, 1973).

Preanaesthetic assessment of these patients should focus on

cardiorespiratory function. Paretic animals may be dehydrated or have atelectatic lung fields resulting from inability to ambulate. Patient rehydration should be accomplished using balanced electrolyte solutions. Dextrose-containing solutions are contraindicated since they have been shown experimentally to be associated with poorer neurological outcome following spinal ischaemia (Drummond and Moore, 1989).

Patients with spinal lesions, especially those cranial to the thoracolumbar junction, often have impaired autonomic function due to interruption of sympathetic outflow tracts and this often results in decreased cardiovascular reserve, hypotension and bradydysrhythmias (Bendo, Giffin and Cottrell, 1986). A recent study of 85 dogs undergoing cervical spinal decompressive surgery showed a relatively high incidence of intraoperative and early postoperative mortality associated with cardiovascular collapse and respiratory failure (Clark, 1986). Cardiopulmonary function should be monitored carefully in these patients throughout surgery and into the early postoperative period.

Since patients with spinal cord injury are likely to be in pain and often show bradydyshrhythmias, premedication with opioid analgesics, such as pethidine (3–5 mg kg^{-1} i.m.) or butorphanol (0.1–0.2 mg kg^{-1} i.m.), and an anticholinergic agent is beneficial. Profound sedation is contraindicated, especially in animals with traumatic spinal injuries, since this may decrease muscle tone and remove the protective splinting effect of the epaxial musculature. If a myelogram is planned, then the interaction of anaesthetic agents and postmyelogram seizures should be taken into account.

Induction of anaesthesia should be rapid and smooth to avoid patient struggling which could adversely affect the lesion. Intravenous induction with a thiobarbiturate, such as thiopentone, is suited to this purpose and may protect neural tissue from further ischaemic damage.

Intubation is best performed by direct vision using a laryngoscope. Where cervical lesions are present or suspected (as in the case of fractures or luxations) the head and neck should be held rigid in relation to the body, preferably by an assistant, to facilitate atraumatic intubation. Great care is needed when moving or positioning patients with spinal lesions to avoid further damage (Gilroy, 1985).

Anaesthesia should be maintained with adequate levels of a volatile anaesthetic agent. Light anaesthesia should be avoided because any movement of the animal is potentially hazardous during neurosurgery and because inadequate levels of anaesthesia may exacerbate pre-existent deleterious autonomic responses. The use of neuromuscular relaxants is often beneficial in these patients.

The electrocardiogram and arterial pressure should be closely monitored because of the likelihood of bradydysrhythmias and hypotension during surgery. Bradycardia may result from the spinal lesion itself or as a result of direct vagal stimulation when a ventral cervical surgical approach is used. Sinus bradycardia and atrioventricular blocks should be treated with atropine (0.02–0.06 mg kg^{-1} i.v.). Hypotension will usually respond to crystalloid or colloid administration. A significant volume of blood may be lost if a vertebral venous sinus is ruptured during surgery. Loss of more than 20% of blood volume requires replacement with either whole blood or packed cells.

Respiratory function should be closely monitored especially in animals with a cervical lesion (Clark, 1986). Hypoventilation or respiratory arrest in these patients may result from the spinal lesion or from obstruction of the airway by excessive tracheal traction during a ventral surgical approach. A wire reinforced endotracheal tube should be used in these patients to decrease the likelihood of iatrogenic obstruction.

Neurological and cardiorespiratory function should be closely monitored during the immediate postoperative period. These patients often experience considerable pain and discomfort resulting in a stormy, vocal recovery with concurrent signs of sympathetic activation. Analgesics, such as butorphanol (0.1–0.4 mg kg^{-1} i.m.) or morphine 0.2–0.5 mg kg^{-1} i.m.), and sedatives or muscle relaxants, such as acepromazine (0.025–0.05 mg kg^{-1} i.m.) or diazepam (0.1–0.4 mg kg^{-1} i.m.), are indicated. If myelography was performed, then the animal should be closely monitored for seizures and treated as necessary with diazepam (0.1–0.4 mg kg^{-1} i.v.).

NEURODIAGNOSTIC PROCEDURES

Cerebrospinal fluid collection

Cerebrospinal fluid (CSF) collection and laboratory evaluation is frequently performed in veterinary patients as part of a neurodiagnostic work-up. In small animal patients, the tap is usually performed at the level of the cisterna magna during general anaesthesia. CSF pressure measurements using a manometer are usually performed during CSF collection to determine where the patient lies on the intracranial compliance curve. Because of the varying effects of anaesthetic technique on CSF pressure, anaesthetic agents, in addition to the position of the patient, and method of measurement should be standardized between patients (Shores *et al.*, 1985).

Preanaesthetic evaluation of these patients should attempt to detect the presence of intracranial hypertension. Removal of CSF through the cisterna magna in patients with increased intracranial pressure may result in herniation of the brain through the foramen magnum. Animals with obvious signs of intracranial hypertension should be treated with mannitol or frusemide before anaesthesia to reduce the risk of herniation.

Anaesthetic agents should be selected which reduce or at least minimize alterations in intracranial pressure. An opioid agent, such as pethidine or butorphanol, with or without a benzodiazepine, such as diazepam, is usually sufficient for premedication. Occasionally, patients are sufficiently obtunded that a premedicant is not required. The agent of choice for induction is an ultrashort-acting thiobarbiturate. Since extreme flexion of the neck during CSF collection may result in occlusion of the airway, all patients should be intubated with a non-collapsible endotracheal tube. These procedures may take less than 15 minutes. Therefore it may be possible to complete the procedure solely under intravenous anaesthesia. If the procedure is anticipated to be longer in duration, then anaesthesia should be maintained using an inhalational anaesthestic such as isoflurane.

Heart rate and ventilatory parameters should be closely monitored during and immediately following CSF collection (Gilroy, 1985). Transient apnoea may result from occlusion of the airway during excessive flexion of the neck especially if a standard endotracheal tube is used. Sustained apnoea may indicate iatrogenic trauma (pithing) or brain herniation. Bradydysrhythmias may also be observed in these patients associated with stimulation of carotid baroreceptors or vagal irritation during neck flexion. These dysrhythmias usually respond to neck extension or atropine.

Myelography

Myelography is a useful tool in small animal practice for the diagnosis of compressive spinal cord disease. This procedure involves injection of a radiopaque agent, usually metrizamide, iopamidol or iohexol, into the subarachnoid space at the level of the cisterna magna or lumbar spine. Radiographs are then taken to define areas of compression as identified by tapering or loss of th dye column.

Complications of myelography which relate to anaesthesia include cardiopulmonary abnormalities and seizures (Dennis and Herrtage, 1987). Transient apnoea or tachypnoea, bradycardia or tachycardia, and hypotension or hypertension have been reported to occur during or immediately following dye injection. These complications are minimized by ensuring an adequate anaesthetic depth before injection, by warming the contrast agent to body temperature and by injecting slowly at a steady rate. Heart rate, blood pressure and respiration should be closely monitored during this period and abnormalities treated accordingly (Gilroy, 1985).

Seizures, after myelography, occur during the recovery period with a reported frequency of 15–50% (Gray, Indrieri and Lippert, 1987). Factors which have been suggested to influence the incidence of postmyelographic seizures include the volume of agent injected, rate of injection, body weight, site of injection, pH of the agent, duration of anaesthesia after completion of the myelogram and patient position after injection (Dennis and Herrtage, 1987). The frequency of seizures has been shown to be increased in dogs which weigh over 25 kg and when the cisternal site as opposed to a lumbar site is used for injection of the dye. Procedures which may minimize seizure incidence therefore include basing dosage on body surface area rather than on body weight, limiting the speed of injection, using the lumbar site where possible, and elevating the patient's head immediately following a cisternal injection to avoid cranial flow of the agent (Shores and Burns, 1987).

Recently, it has been shown that the choice of anaesthetic drugs and intravenous fluids influences the incidence of seizures after myelography. Dogs that were premedicated with phenobarbitone or pentobarbitone and maintained on methoxyflurane had a lower incidence of seizures than those anaesthetized without barbiturate premedication or with halothane (Gray, Indrieri and Lippert, 1987). This effect may in part result from the prolongation of recovery from anaesthesia by using both barbiturates and methoxyflurane in the anaesthetic protocol. It has also been demonstrated that intravenous infusion of a 5% dextrose in water solution over the course of the procedure greatly reduces the incidence of metrizamide-induced seizures (Gray, Lowrie and Wetmore, 1987; Tamas, Walker and Paddleford, 1986). This may be explained by the fact that metrizamide is a competitive inhibitor of brain hexokinase, and therefore may induce a degree of neuroglucopenia. The administration of dextrose solutions can overcome this effect. It should be remembered, however, that dextrose solutions may promote CNS oedema formation and decrease local tissue pH by being metabolized to form water and acid byproducts. For these reasons, dextrose-containing solutions are contraindicated for use in patients with ischaemic lesions. It is unlikely that dextrose administration during iopamidol or iohexol myelography would reduce the incidence of postmyelographic seizures since these agents do not affect glucose metabolism. Use of these newer agents appears to be associated with a lower incidence of postmyelographic seizures than with metrizamide (Dennis and Herrtage, 1987).

Based on the preceding observations, an appropriate anaesthetic regimen for patients undergoing myelography would include premedication with phenobarbitone (2 mg kg^{-1} i.m.) or pentobarbitone (5 mg kg^{-1} i.m.), induction with a thiobarbiturate and maintenance with methoxyflurane. Anaesthesia should be maintained for at least 60 minutes following injection of the dye and the animal should be positioned with the head elevated above the body to decrease rostral spread of the contrast media. The patient should be monitored closely immediately following injection of the dye for adverse cardiopulmonary effects and also during recovery for the development of seizures. Therapy for postmyelographic seizures consists of intravenous diazepam (0.1–0.4 mg kg^{-1}) or if the patient is refractory to this drug, phenobarbitone (2–4 mg kg^{-1} i.v.) may be administered (Shores and Burns, 1987).

REFERENCES

Albin, M. S., White, R. J. and Acosta-Rua, G. (1968). *Journal of Neurosurgery* **29**, 113.

Bendo, A. A., Griffin, J. P. and Cottrell, J. E. (1986). In *Anesthesia and Neurosurgery*, 2nd edn, p. 392. St Louis, Missouri: The C.V. Mosby Co.

Bennett, D. R., Madsen, J. A. and Jordan, W. S. (1973). *Neurology* **23**, 449.

Braund, K. G. (1987). In *Veterinary Neurology*, eds. J. E. Oliver, B. F. Hoerlein & I. G. Mayhew, p. 278. Philadelphia: W. B. Saunders Co.

Brown, R. S., Mohr, P. A. and Carey, J. J. (1967). *Surgery, Gynecology and Obstetrics* **125**, 1205.

Bruce, D. A. (1986). In *Anesthesia and Neurosurgery*, 2nd edn, p. 150. St Louis, Missouri: The C. V. Mosby Co.

Clark, D. M. (1986). *Journal of the American Animal Hospital Association* **22**, 739.

Cottrell, J. E., Robustelli, A., Post, K. and Turndorf, H. (1977). *Anesthesiology* **47**, 28.

Court, M. H., Dodman, N. H., Norman, W. M. and Seeler, D. C. (1988). *British Veterinary Journal* **144**, 323.

Dennis, R. and Herrtage, M. E. (1987). *Veterinary Radiology* **30**, 2.

Drummond, J. C. and Moore, S. S. (1989). *Anesthesiology* **70**, 64.

Dyson, D. H. (1988). *Journal of the American Medical Association* **192**, 1286.

Faden, A. I., Jacobs, T. P. and Holaday, J. W. (1981). *Science* **211**, 493.

Faden, A. I., Jacobs, T. P., Mougey, E. and Holaday, J. W. (1981). *Annals of Neurology* **10**, 326.

Fankhauser, R., Luginbuhl, H. and McGrath, J. T. (1974). *Bulletin of the World Health Organization* **50**, 53

Fenner, W. R. (1986). In *Current Veterinary Therapy IX. Small Animal Practice*, ed. R. W. Kirk, p. 830. Philadelphia: W. B. Saunders Co.

Frost, E. A. M. (1986). *37th Annual Refresher Courses of the ASA*, 124.

Gilroy, B. A. (1984). In *Textbook of Small Animal Surgery*, ed. D. H. Slatter, p. 2643. Philadelphia: W. B. Saunders Co.

Gilroy, B. A. and Anson, L. W. (1987). *Journal of the American Veterinary Association* **190**, 552.

Gray, P. R., Lowrie, C. T. and Wetmore, L. A. (1987). *American Journal of Veterinary Research* **48**, 1600.

Hamill, J. F., Bedford, R. F. and Weaver, D. C. (1981). *Anesthesiology* **55**, 578.

Hartzog, J. T., Fischer, R. G. and Snow, C. (1971). In *Proceedings of the Veteran's Administration Spinal Cord Injury Conference* **17**, 70.

Hayes, K. C. and Schiefer, B. (1969). *Pathologica Veterinaria* **6**, 94.

Indrieri, R. J. and Simpson, S. T. (1985). In *Textbook of Small Animal Surgery*, ed. D. H. Slatter, p. 1415. Philadelphia; W. B. Saunders Co.

Kajihara, K., Kawanaga, H. and de la Torre, J. C. (1973). *Surgery and Neurology* **1**, 16.

Kobrine, A. I., Doyle, T. F. and Martins, A. N. (1975). *Journal of Neurosurgery* **42**, 144.

Kolata, R. J., Kraut, N. H. and Johnston, D. L. (1974). *Journal of the American Medical Association* **164**, 499.

Kornegay, J. N. (1985). In *Textbook of Small Animal Surgery*, ed. D. H. Slatter, p. 1266. Philadelphia: W. B. Saunders Co.

Lassen, N. A. (1966). *Lancet* **ii**, 113.

LeCouteur, R. A. and Turrel, J. M. (1986). In *Current Veterinary Therapy IX, Small Animal Practice*, ed. R. W. Kirk, p. 820. Philadelphia: W. B. Saunders Co.

Matjasko, M. J. (1986). In *Anesthesia and Neurosurgery*, 2nd edn, p. 188. St Louis, Missouri: The C. V. Mosby Co.

Michenfelder, J. D. (1983). In *Complications in Anesthesiology*, eds. F. K. Orkin and L. H. Cooperman, p. 268. Philadelphia: J. B. Lippincott.

Miner, M. E. and Allen, S. J. (1984). In *Clinical Anesthesia in Neurosurgery*, ed. E. A. M. Frost, p. 367. Boston: Butterworths.

Moorthy, S. S. and Hilgenberg, J. C. (1980). *Anesthesia and Analgesia*

59, 131.

Nafe, L. A. (1979). *Journal of the American Veterinary Medical Association* **174**, 1224.

Rosa, G., Orfei, P. and Sanfilippo, M. (1986). *Anesthesia and Analgesia* **65**, 381.

Rosa, G., Sanfilippo, M. and Vilardi, V. (1986). *Anesthesia and Analgesia* **58**, 437.

Rucker, N. C., Lumb, W. V. and Scott, R. J. (1981). *American Journal of Veterinary Research* **42**, 1138.

Samuels, S. I. (1986). In *Anesthesia and Neurosurgery*, 2nd edn, p. 114. St Louis, Missouri: The C. V. Mosby Co.

Shores, A., Braund, K. G., Stockham, S. L. and Simpson, S. T. (1985). In *Textbook of Small Animal Surgery*, ed. D. H. Slatter, p. 1285. Philadelphia: W. B. Saunders Co.

Shores, A. and Burns, J. (1987). *The Compendium on Continuing Education for the Practicing Veterinarian* **9**, 361.

Stoelting, R. K., Dierdorf, S. F. and McCammon, R. L. (1988). In *Anesthesia and Co-Existing Disease*, 2nd edn, p. 263. New York: Churchill Livingstone.

Tamas, P. M., Walker, M. A. and Paddleford, R. R. (1986). *Journal of the American Veterinary Medical Association* **188**, 710.

Turrel, J. M., Fike, J. R. and LeCouteur, R. A. (1984). *Journal of the American Veterinary Medical Association* **184**, 82.

Walker, T. L. and Betts, C. W. (1985). In *Textbook of Small Animal Surgery*, ed. D. H. Slatter, p. 1396. Philadelphia: W. B. Saunders Co.

Walker, T. L., Tomlinson, J., Sorjonen, D. C. and Kornegay, J. N. (1985). In *Textbook of Small Animal Surgery*, ed. D. H. Slatter, p. 1367. Philadelphia: W. B. Saunders Co.

12

Anaesthesia for patients with neuromuscular disease

Diseases resulting in disturbances of neural, neuromuscular or muscular function, although rare and often obscure, may be associated with life-threatening perioperative complications, such as respiratory and cardiac decompensation. The clinical presentation, neurodiagnostic responses and pathophysiological mechanisms involved in these conditions are discussed elsewhere (Chrisman and Averill, 1983; Craig, 1989; DeLahunta, 1983; Kortz, 1989; Lecouteur, Dow and Sisson, 1989; Luttgen, 1989; Sharp, Kornegay and Lane, 1989; Smith, 1989). Patients with these conditions may not respond as expected to anaesthetic agents and adjuncts. The following discussion will focus on selecting anaesthetic techniques appropriate for small animals with peripheral neuropathy, diseases of the neuromuscular junction or with myopathy.

PHYSIOLOGY OF NEUROMUSCULAR TRANSMISSION

Skeletal muscles are controlled by myelinated nerve fibres originating from the ventral motor neurons located in the spinal cord grey matter. These nerve fibres have multiple branches and can innervate numerous muscle fibres. The neuromuscular junction is the point where the nerve invaginates into the muscle fibre and is separated from the muscle by a gap termed the junctional or synaptic cleft. Corrugations in the muscle membrane (subneural clefts) increase the surface area where the neurotransmitter, acetylcholine (ACh), acts. Vesicles storing ACh are located in the axon terminals. A nerve impulse, by decreasing membrane potential, causes an influx of Ca^{2+} into the nerve terminal and subsequently induces release of ACh from the synaptic vesicles. After liberation from the synaptic vesicles, ACh binds to postsynaptic ACh receptors causing a rapid influx of Na^+ into the muscle fibre and local depolarization of the motor end plate. This end plate potential, if of sufficient magnitude, results in a propagated muscle action potential. Depolarization of the sarcolemma stimulates release of Ca^{2+} stores from the sarcoplasmic reticulum causing activation of the excitation–contraction coupling process. The net result of this process is muscular contraction. ACh is rapidly hydrolysed by the enzyme, acetylcholinesterase (AChE), and repolarization of the sarcolemma occurs (Guyton, 1986).

ANAESTHETIC CONSIDERATIONS

Peripheral neuropathy

The peripheral neuropathies, associated pathophysiology and selected diagnostic criteria are given in Table 1.

Preoperative evaluation. The effect of peripheral neuropathies on respiratory function is a primary concern during anaesthesia. Muscle weakness, which is associated with these conditions, will reduce the functional residual capacity and depress alveolar ventilation. Respiratory function should always be evaluated carefully prior to anaesthesia. A description of the preoperative assessment of respiratory function has been provided by Dodman *et al.* (1987). Other complications of peripheral neuropathies include laryngeal paralysis, paraesthesias and regurgitation. Patients that regurgitate may develop aspiration pneumonia which will further compromise respiratory function.

In order to decrease the risks associated with general anaesthesia, the condition of the patient should be improved before anaesthesia when possible by medical intervention. Postponement of surgery and anaesthesia is prudent in those cases likely to improve with specific therapy (e.g. diabetic neuropathy in cats) or when spontaneous recovery may occur (e.g. idiopathic neuropathy, post-rabies vaccination polyneuropathy). Secondary complications should also be treated as far as possible prior to anaesthesia. There will be times, however, when a delay is not possible or is unlikely to improve the anaesthetic risk to the patient. In these cases it will be necessary to proceed with caution in the face of adversity.

Premedication. When respiratory compromise is present, preanaesthetics, such as acepromazine, which produce mild sedation with minimal respiratory depression are most appropriate. The benzodiazepine tranquillizers, midazolam or diazepam, may also be useful. These agents cause minimal cardiorespiratory depression. However, dysphoria rather than sedation may occur

Table 1. Clinical features of peripheral neuropathies affecting small animal patients

Disease	Pathophysiology	Clinical signs	Breeds	Diagnosis
Idiopathic polyneuropathies:				
Idiopathic polyradiculoneuritis (coonhound paralysis)	Demyelination of ventral spinal root	Progressive weakness Hypotonic or atonic Voice weakness Hyperaesthesia	Any breed	EMG Clinical signs
Distal denervating disease	Diffuse degeneration of axonal myelin	Similar to above No hyperaesthesia	Any breed	EMG Clinical signs
Familial polyneuropathies:				
Inherited hypertrophic neuropathy in Tibetan Mastiffs	Demyelination and Schwann cell hyperplasia of peripheral nerves	Progressive weakness at 7–12 weeks of age	Tibetan Mastiffs	EMG Clinical signs
Giant axonal neuropathy	Peripheral axonal swelling and demyelination	Progressive pelvic limb paresis Voice weakness Regurgitation	German Shepherds	EMG Clinical signs
Progressive spinal muscular atrophy	Abiotrophy of ventral horn cells	Progressive weakness at 5–7 weeks	Swedish Lapland Britanny Spaniels	
Globoid cell leukodystrophy	Widespread demyelination	Progressive weakness at 4–6 months	West Highland Terriers Cairn Terriers	β-galactocerebrosidase assay

Table 1. *Continued*

Disease	Pathophysiology	Clinical signs	Breeds	Diagnosis
Metabolic polyneuropathies: Diabetes mellitus Hyperinsulinaemia Hypothyroidism Chronic renal failure Cushing's syndrome	Related to metabolic disorder	Quadriparesis or quadriplegia Depressed spinal reflexes	Any breed	EMG Clinical signs Peripheral nerve biopsy
Immune-mediated polyneuropathies: Systemic lupus erythematosus	Related to auto antibody formulation	Generalized weakness Depressed spinal reflexes	Any breed	EMG Clinical signs SLE assay
Post-rabies vaccination polyneuropathy	Unknown	Ascending flaccid quadriplegia 7–10 days after rabies vaccination	Any breed	History Clinical signs EMG

in some patients. The α_2-agonists, xylazine and medetomidine, and the opioid agonists are dose-dependent respiratory depressants and should be used with caution in patients with ventilatory impairment. These agents may also induce vomition which could predispose to aspiration pneumonia, particularly in animals with laryngeal paralysis. If opioids are to be used, the agonist–antagonists have the advantage of providing mild sedation and analgesia with only minimal changes in cardiorespiratory function. Neuroleptanalgesic combinations, such as droperidol/ fentanyl or acepromazine/oxymorphone, are reasonably safe because sedation can be achieved with lower doses of each drug thereby minimizing adverse effects.

Anticholinergics (atropine or glycopyrronium), if indicated, may be safely administered to patients with peripheral neuropathies. Oxygen supplementation via face mask or nasal tube prior to induction is beneficial in those patients with existing respiratory compromise.

Induction. Rapid control of the airway is extremely important in those animals with ventilatory disturbance and can best be achieved by the intravenous administration of an ultrashort-acting barbiturate. Barbiturates should be administered incrementally until intubation is possible. Maintenance of a patent airway with a snug-fitting cuffed endotracheal tube is recommended and will facilitate intermittent positive pressure ventilation (IPPV) of the lungs. Opioid agonists, such as oxymorphone, may be used safely for induction of anaesthesia. These agents have the advantage that they can be effectively antagonized by specific opioid antagonists, if necessary. Dissociative anaesthetics are best avoided in dogs as they may induce excitement and convulsions during recovery. Induction with inhalation agents is safe, but may be prolonged in patients with ventilatory disturbances.

Maintenance. Anaesthesia should be maintained with either isoflurane or halothane. These agents have relatively low blood solubility which facilitates rapid induction and recovery. Nitrous oxide should be used with caution if respiratory depression is detected preoperatively. Human patients with Guillain–Barré syndrome, which is very similar to canine idiopathic polyradiculoneuritis, may have a pronounced rise in serum potassium following the administration of depolarizing muscle relaxants (Dierdorf, 1989). Excessive release of potassium and resultant ventricular fibrillation have also been associated with the administration of suxamethonium (succinylcholine) to human patients with denervation injuries (Griffin, 1984). If relaxants are to be used as part of the anaesthetic protocol, non-depolarizing agents, such as atracurium and vecuronium, are effective and safe alternatives to suxamethonium.

Humans with Guillain–Barré syndrome often have autonomic dysfunction which may induce profound changes in blood pressure and heart rate. These changes have been reported to cause cardiac dysrhythmias and even cardiac arrest (Krone, Reuther and Fuhrmeister, 1983). In addition, autonomic compensatory responses to changes in cardiovascular status may be impaired, leading to significant hypotension during moderate hypovolaemia or IPPV (Dierdorf, 1989). It is also reported that surgical stimulation of these patients may cause unexpected tachycardia, hypertension and cardiac dysrhythmias (Moore and James, 1981). Similar considerations may apply to small animal patients with demyelinating neuropathies. In these cases, the cardiovascular system should be closely monitored so that disturbances may be detected and treated early. Vasodilator or vasoconstrictor therapy may be indicated.

Careful attention should be paid to the ventilatory status of the patients with moderate to severe neuropathies. Routine monitoring of tidal and minute ventilation (via Wright's respirometer), mucous membrane colour and the electrocardiogram may alert the clinician to impending complications. Arterial blood gas analysis, if available, will provide the most definitive information about ventilation. Intermittent positive pressure ventilation should be initiated if muscle relaxants are used or if spontaneous ventilation is inadequate.

Recovery. Close supervision of the patient is imperative during the recovery period. It is advisable to leave the endotracheal tube in place with the cuff inflated until laryngeal and pharyngeal reflexes have returned. If regurgitation occurs, the oral cavity should be lavaged with water and the endotracheal tube removed with the cuff inflated to decrease the likelihood of aspiration. The ventilatory status of the patient should be evaluated regularly and supplementary oxygen should be administered if necessary. When significant respiratory depression is detected, mechanical ventilation may have to be initiated. If opioids or non-depolarizing muscle relaxants are the cause of respiratory depression, they should be reversed with their respective antagonists.

Small animals with demyelinating neuropathies are sometimes hyperaesthetic to sensory stimuli and would benefit from analgesic therapy. Opioid agonist–antagonists, such as butorphanol, provide effective analgesia with minimal respiratory depression. Pure opioid agonists are also useful provided that large dosages are avoided. It has been suggested that human patients with Guillain–Barré syndrome should receive epidural opioids since this form of analgesic therapy provides effective pain relief with minimal respiratory depression (Rosenfeld, Borel and Hanley, 1986). Epidural opioid analgesia may offer similar advantages for small animal patients with peripheral neuropathy.

Diseases affecting the neuromuscular junction.

Diseases of the neuromuscular junction are of concern to the anaesthetist primarily because of their effects on the muscles of respiration. The mechanism of the impairment, however, is quite different from that of the neuropathies (dealt with above) and the anaesthetic management of these cases requires a somewhat different approach. Disorders of the neuromuscular junction, their pathophysiology and clinical signs are listed in Table 2.

Preoperative evaluation. The clinical history should be elicited from the owner and a physical examination and routine laboratory tests should be performed (Dodman, Seeler and Court, 1984). Additional tests to determine the presence and degree of ventilatory dysfunction are indicated in moderately to severely affected animals (Dodman *et al.*, 1987). Information relating to generalized weakness, exercise intolerance and post-exertional muscle weakness is particularly helpful in evaluating the severity of the condition. The owner should be questioned about any changes in the animal's voice as this may indicate laryngeal dysfunction. The ability of the animal to swallow should also be elucidated by questioning and by observation. Incidents of regurgitation following eating may indicate megaoesophagus in myasthenic patients. This should be further investigated radiographically using positive contrast if necessary. Megaoesophagus is present in most but not all dogs with myasthenia gravis (Shelton, 1989). Preoperative chest radiographs are desirable in myasthenic patients to evaluate the lungs for evidence of aspiration pneumonia and to determine the presence or absence of a thymoma. Thymoma associated with myasthenia gravis can occur in a small percentage of older dogs (Shelton, 1989). Myasthenic dogs may be better candidates for anaesthesia if they are treated with long-acting anticholinesterase drugs. The response to therapy can be good, leading to rapid remission of clinical signs of muscle weakness. Megaoesophagus may also resolve but this takes longer (Shelton, 1989). Animals with tick paralysis, botulism or organophosphorus (anticholinesterase) toxicosis should not be anaesthetized except for emergency procedures. In these cases, symptomatic therapy is valuable preoperatively but specific therapeutic manoeuvres are also indicated.

Table 2. Clinical features of diseases of the neuromuscular junction

Disease	Pathophysiology	Clinical signs	Breed	Diagnosis
Acquired myasthenia gravis	Autoantibodies against postsynaptic nicotinic ACh receptors	Post-exertional muscle weakness Megaoesophagus Laryngeal and/or pharyngeal weakness Thymoma	German Shepherd Golden Retrievers	Alleviation of weakness after edrophonium chloride EMG Autoantibodies
Congenital myasthenia	Deficiency in muscle ACh receptors	Post-exertional muscle weakness Megaoesophagus Laryngeal and/or pharyngeal weakness Thymoma	Jack Russell Terrier Springer Spaniel Smooth Fox Terrier	Similar to above but no autoantibodies
Tick paralysis	Neurotoxin prevents normal release of ACh	Generalized weakness Death from respiratory paralysis	Any breed	EMG Clinical signs Tick detection
Botulism	Botulism toxin blocks release of ACh from cholinergic nerve terminals	Rapid paralysis progressing from pelvic limbs to thoracic limbs Dysphagia Regurgitation Hyporeflexia	Any breed	EMG Toxin in serum and faeces
Acetylcholinesterase inhibiting insecticides	Binds AChE	Salivation Lacrimation Diarrhoea Muscle tremors Respiratory paralysis	Any breed	AChE assay Clinical signs

Premedication. The use of preoperative sedatives and opioids should be curtailed in patients with myasthenia gravis because of the potential for intraoperative or postoperative respiratory failure. Acepromazine at doses of less than 0.05 mg kg^{-1} i.m. is normally safe. Xylazine and medetomidine are not recommended for premedication of patients with respiratory depression or laryngeal/pharyngeal dysfunction. If opioids are required, then agents with mixed agonist/antagonist activity, such as butorphanol, may be more appropriate.

Anticholinergics are particularly desirable in patients on anticholinesterase therapy as these patients may have increased vagal responsiveness and are prone to develop bradycardia (McLeod and Creighton, 1986). The use of anticholinergic premedication is imperative in cases of anticholinesterase intoxication.

Induction. Preoxygenation, by allowing the patient to breathe pure oxygen for 3–5 minutes before induction, is advisable to offset hypoxia secondary to hypoventilation and ventilation–perfusion mismatch. Anaesthesia can then be induced safely with thiopentone, administered intravenously at a dose sufficient to relax the jaw and obtund the swallowing reflex. During induction, the head should be held higher than the body to prevent passive reflux of material from the oesophagus into the pharynx. A well-fitting endotracheal tube should be inserted following induction of anaesthesia and the cuff should be inflated before the animal's head is lowered.

Other anaesthetic induction techniques offer no definite advantage over thiopentone in otherwise healthy patients. In cats, alphaxalone/alphadolone acetate may be used for induction of anaesthesia unless there is a history of hypersensitivity to this steroid anaesthetic. Dissociative anaesthetics are also acceptable induction agents in cats, but use in dogs is associated with an unacceptable incidence of postanaesthetic excitement and seizure activity. Induction of anaesthesia with high doses of opioids (administered i.v.) may be the preferred method of induction in dogs when thiobarbiturates are contraindicated. Opioids are readily reversible with specific antagonists, and respiratory depression following anaesthetic induction may be managed by means of IPPV. Induction of anaesthesia by inhalation is not recommended for patients with megaoesophagus because of an increased risk of passive regurgitation and subsequent aspiration of oesophageal contents.

Maintenance of anaesthesia. Isoflurane and halothane are suitable agents for the maintenance of anaesthesia in these patients. Nitrous oxide may be used to supplement either anaesthetic agent and thus reduce their requirement, but if this is done, care should be taken to avoid hypoxaemia. Nitrous oxide should be avoided during thoracotomy (e.g. for thymectomy) because packing off the lungs to facilitate surgical access will increase the risk of hypoxaemia. Also, diffusion of nitrous oxide into any residual postsurgical pneumothorax can be a problem unless the patient is receiving continuous chest drainage.

A major concern during maintenance of anaesthesia is whether ventilation is adequate. The simplest way to check for ventilatory adequacy is with a respirometer. Blood gas analysis is the definitive test of the adequacy of ventilation but facilities for this may not be available in veterinary practice.

Should the use of muscle relaxants be contemplated as part of a maximal support maintenance technique (balanced anaesthesia), it should be noted that patients with myasthenic conditions exhibit increased sensitivity to non-depolarizing muscle relaxants (Smith, Donati and Bevan, 1989). The response to depolarizing blockers is also unpredictable, sometimes resulting in a prolonged ('dual') block (McLeod and Creighton, 1986). Neuromuscular blocking agents are often avoided in myasthenic human patients because of their unpredictable response (Pollard, Harper and Doran, 1989). If muscle relaxants are desired, it is probably better to use a non-depolarizing blocker and to titrate the dose carefully to produce the desired effect. Atracurium appears to be the relaxant of choice because of rapid spontaneous breakdown (McLeod and Creighton, 1986). The potency of atracurium is increased by a factor of 1.7–1.9 in myasthenia gravis (Smith *et al.*, 1989). Thus reduced doses should be adequate to produce the requisite degree of relaxation. The myasthenic patient can be thought of as partially blocked at the neuromuscular junction prior to the administration of the non-depolarizing drug. Once recovery from atracurium starts, the time to full return of neuromuscular function is not prolonged in myasthenic patients (Smith *et al.*, 1989). Intermittent positive pressure ventilation of the lungs is mandatory when muscle relaxants are employed. Care must be exercised to maintain the unconscious state in paralysed patients.

Recovery. There are two main considerations when recovering animals with neuromuscular disease. The first concerns the airway, its reflex activity, patency and the possibility of aspiration of oesophageal or stomach contents. This concern may be addressed by leaving the endotracheal tube in longer than normal with the cuff inflated and by carefully assessing the return of laryngeal and pharyngeal reflexes prior to extubation. The second major concern is the postoperative establishment and maintenance of adequate pulmonary ventilation. As previously mentioned, use of a respirometer or blood gas analysis is valuable in this situation. If ventilation is inadequate, the inspired air should be supplemented with oxygen and it may be necessary to ventilate the lungs until any residual respiratory depressant effects of anaesthetic agents have dissipated. Some agents, for example, opioids and non-depolarizing muscle relaxants, lend themselves to reversal with specific antagonist drugs.

Postoperative analgesia is an additional concern, especially following thoracotomy where incisional pain may limit effective thoracic excursions. The systemic administration of opioids is often effective for this purpose, but must be viewed with caution because of the potential for profound respiratory depression, especially if large doses are required. An alternative technique for analgesia is to administer opioids epidurally through the lumbosacral space. This has been reported to provide excellent postoperative analgesia in human patients without associated respiratory depression (Keith, Clark and Saint John, 1989). Special preservative-free preparations of the opioids are required for this technique, which is now common practice in all human hospitals and some veterinary hospitals.

Myopathy

Myopathies which have been described in small animal patients and the affected breeds are listed in Table 3.

Preoperative evaluation. Generalized muscle weakness is common to many of the myopathies in small animals. Unfortunately, muscle dysfunction is not limited to the muscles of posture and locomotion, but also affects respiratory, oropharyngeal, laryngeal, oesophageal and occasionally cardiac muscles. Ventilatory insufficiency, dysphagia, megaoesophagus, aspiration pneumonia, cardiomyopathy and associated cardiac rhythm disturbances are clinically important abnormalities that may be detected during preoperative evaluation. Animals with glycogen storage disease may show hepatic dysfunction (Lecouteur, Dow and Sisson, 1989). Apart from routine clinical procedures, preoperative examination of animals with myopathy should include careful auscultation of heart and lungs, thoracic radiographs, electrocardiogram, complete blood count, biochemistry profile, and if cardiomyopathy is suspected, echocardiographic evaluation of heart function. Ventilatory status should be assessed using techniques which have been described previously (Dodman *et al.*, 1987). If pneumonia is detected, affected animals should be treated with appropriate antibiotic therapy prior to elective anaesthesia.

Patients with malignant hyperthermia (MH) or exertional

Table 3. Myopathies affecting small animals

Disease	Breed
Congenital:	
Canine myotonia	Chow Chow
	Staffordshire Bull Terrier
	West Highland White Terrier
	Great Dane
	Labrador Retriever
Golden retriever muscular dystrophy	Golden Retriever
Irish Terrier myopathy	Irish Terrier
Labrador Retriever myopathy	Labrador Retriever
Dystrophy-like myopathy in cats	Domestic short-hair
Metabolic:	
Malignant hyperthermia	Greyhound
Exertional myopathy	Greyhound
Glycogen storage disease	Lapland Dogs
Mitochondrial myopathies	Clumber spaniels
	Sussex Spaniels
Electrolyte disorders:	
Hypo- and hyperkalaemic myopathies	Any breed
Endocrine:	
Hypo- and hyperthyroid myopathies	Any breed
Hypo- and hyperadrenocorticoid myopathies	Any breed
Hypo- and hyperparathyroid myopathies	Any breed
Diabetes mellitus	Any breed
Idiopathic:	
Masticatory myositis	Any breed
Polymyositis	Any breed

myopathy may not demonstrate any abnormalities unless stimulated by appropriate triggering conditions. Such conditions may include stress, exercise or the administration of certain anaesthetic agents. Table 4 lists anaesthetic agents which have been implicated in the pathogenesis of MH. There are no specific diagnostic tests for MH that can be easily applied to small animals. Malignant

Table 4. Anaesthetic agents and adjuncts (triggering agents) which have been implicated in the pathogenesis of malignant hyperthermia (MH) and agents which are considered to be safe for use in MH susceptible patients

Drug type	Triggering agents	Safe agents
Muscle relaxants	Suxamethonium (succinylcholine)	Pancuronium Atracurium Vecuronium
Inhalational anaesthetics	Halothane Methoxyflurane Enflurane Isoflurane Ether	Nitrous oxide
Injectable anaesthetics	Ketamine	Barbiturates Opioids Benzodiazepines Neuroleptanalgesic
Local anaesthetics	Lignocaine Mepivacaine (Carbocaine) Bupivacaine Etidocaine	Procaine Tetracaine

hyperthermia may be suspected in animals that previously experienced a hyperthermic episode in association with clinical signs which are suggestive of MH. There appears to be a familial basis for this disease in dogs (O'Brien *et al.*, 1983). Baseline levels of serum creatine kinase should be obtained before anaesthesia to use for comparison and diagnosis if complications develop during or following anaesthesia. Preoperative preparation of suspected MH patients should include treatment with dantrolene, a skeletal muscle relaxant and specific therapeutic agent for MH. This drug is administered orally at 2–4 mg kg^{-1} divided daily for 2 to 3 days before anaesthesia or, more ideally, 1–2 mg kg^{-1} given intravenously before induction of anaesthesia (Flewellyn *et al.*, 1983; Pandit, Kothary and Cohen, 1979).

Premedication. Heavy sedation is rarely needed in animals with myopathy since they are usually weak and unable to resist physical manipulations. Analgesic premedication may be required if myalgia is evident. Minimal amounts of opioid drugs should be used in animals with cardiac or respiratory compromise.

Anxiolytic agents are highly beneficial in animals with suspect MH to reduce perioperative stress. Acepromazine and droperidol were shown to be protective against a halothane-stimulated MH reaction in a porcine MH model, although at higher dosages than are commonly used in dogs and cats (ED_{50}=1.2 mg kg^{-1} for acepromazine and 0.055 mg kg^{-1} for droperidol; McGrath *et al.*, 1980, (1981). Table 4 lists anaesthetic agents which are unlikely to initiate an MH reaction and are considered safe for use in these patients.

Induction. The choice of induction technique in patients with myopathy will be determined by the presence and degree of cardiac and/or respiratory dysfunction. Anaesthetic management of patients with cardiac and respiratory compromise has been discussed previously (Dodman *et al.*, 1987; Seeler *et al.*, 1988). Animals with moderate to severe myopathy tend to be hypersensitive to the central nervous system depressant effects of anaesthetic agents. In these patients, all anaesthetic drugs should be administered using minimal dosages and titrated carefully to effect.

Animals with megaoesophagus should be induced and intubated rapidly, preferably using an intravenous induction technique to decrease the likelihood of aspiration (see previous section for more detail). Dogs with myopathies involving the muscles of mastication may have trismus or fibrotic contracture resulting in inability to open the mouth sufficiently to allow intubation (Smith, 1989). In these patients, it may be necessary to use mechanical retraction to open the mouth. In severe cases, a tracheotomy may be necessary to establish an airway.

Opioid or barbiturate induction techniques are referred for animals with suspected MH. Ketamine and volatile anaesthetics should not be used in these animals.

Maintenance. Isoflurane is the preferred maintenance agent in animals with cardiac dysrhythmias or depressed cardiac function. This agent also allows precise control of anaesthetic depth and rapid return of protective airway reflexes and respiratory function during recovery.

Volatile inhalational anaesthetics must not be used in suspected MH patients. In these animals, a balanced anaesthetic technique involving a potent opioid (oxymorphone or fentanyl), a benzodiazepine (diazepam or midazolam), nitrous oxide and a nondepolarizing muscle relaxant (atracurium or vecuronium) may be used for maintenance of anaesthesia. Depolarizing relaxants, like suxamethonium, are contraindicated as they are triggering agents for MH. Intravenous infusion of propofol is considered safe for use in MH susceptible patients and may provide sufficient relaxation and analgesia for surgical procedures. Regional anaesthesia using either procaine or tetracaine should be used when the surgical site is amenable to the technique. Lignocaine or other amide local anaesthetics should not be used in these patients since they have been shown to be triggering agents for MH. Spinal anaesthesia should be considered for pelvic limb, urogenital or rectal procedures.

Muscle relaxants should be avoided in most patients with myopathy. Depolarizing relaxants result in prolonged muscle contraction in patients with myotonia (Mitchell, Ali and Savarese, 1978). Non-depolarizing relaxants may have an exaggerated effect in animals with muscle weakness as a result of myopathy. Reversal of neuromuscular blockade using anticholinesterase drugs, such as neostigmine and edrophonium, would be expected to induce excessive and prolonged muscular spasm in patients with myotonia. At least in two cases of myotonia in human patients, this did not occur when neostigmine was used (Ravin, Newmark and Saviello, 1975). Careful titration of a predictable, intermediate-acting relaxant, such as atracurium, may obviate the need for pharmacological reversal in selected cases.

The electrocardiogram, blood pressure and adequacy of ventilation should be monitored in patients with myopathy. Those that show evidence of respiratory failure should be mechanically ventilated. Body temperature should also be monitored frequently, preferably continuously with a thermistor, in myotonic and MH susceptible patients since these animals are prone to becoming hyperthermic during anaesthesia. Hypothermia should be avoided since postoperative shivering may stimulate mytonia in susceptible patients. Table 5 lists clinical signs associated with development of a fulminant MH reaction. An emergency treatment protocol for an MH reaction is summarized in Table 6.

Table 5. Clinical signs associated with development of a fulminant malignant hyperthermia reaction

---

Tachycardia (sudden, unexplained)
Tachypnoea
Cardiac dysrhythmias
Unstable blood pressure
Temperature increase (1 °C every 15 min to 43 °C or higher)
Muscle fasciculations/rigidity
Soda lime becomes hotter than usual and changes colour quickly
Arterial blood gas shows hypoxia, metabolic and respiratory acidosis
Hyperkalaemia
Myoglobinuria (late)
Elevated creatine kinase (late)

Table 6. Emergency protocol for treatment of a malignant hyperthermia reaction during anaesthesia

---

1. Stop anaesthesia and surgery immediately
2. Change anaesthetic circuit and soda lime (if possible)
3. Hyperventilate with 100% oxygen
4. Dantrolene 1–2 mg kg^{-1} i.v. up to 10 mg kg^{-1} (2.5 mg kg^{-1} usually effective)
5. Treat cardiac dysrhythmias with procainamide (5–20 mg kg^{-1} i.v. slow)
6. Cool patient vigorously
7. Sodium bicarbonate (1–2 meq kg^{-1} i.v. increments) to correct acidosis and hyperkalaemia
8. Maintain urinary function and treat with mannitol or frusemide if necessary
9. Monitor patient until danger of subsequent episodes has passed
10. Give oral dantrolene during postoperative period

Recovery. Intensive monitoring of cardiorespiratory function should continue into the postoperative period. In particular, these patients are prone to postoperative respiratory failure and may require mechanical ventilation until fully recovered. Animals may develop MH reactions up to 48 hours following anaesthesia. Anaesthetic recovery and postoperative care should therefore be as stress-free as possible in susceptible animals. As previously discussed, postoperative analgesic therapy is recommended for these patients.

REFERENCES

Chrisman, C. L. and Averill, D. R. (1983). In *Textbook of Veterinary Internal Medicine*, 2nd edn, ed. S. J. Ettinger, p. 608, Philadelphia: Saunders.

Craig, T. M. (1989). *Seminars in Veterinary Medicine and Surgery (Small Animal)* **4**, 161.

DeLahunta, A. (1983). In *Veterinary Neuroanatomy and Clinical Neurology*, 2nd ed, p. 53. Philadelphia: Saunders.

Dierdorf, S. F. (1989). In *Clinical Anesthesia*, eds. P. G. Barash, B. F. Cohen & R. K. Stoelting, p. 443. Philadelphia: J. B. Lippincott.

Dodman, N. H., Seeler, D. C. and Court, M. H. (1984). *British Journal of Anaesthesia* **140**, 505.

Dodman, N. H., Seeler, D. C., Norman, W. M. and Court, M. H. (1987). *British Veterinary Journal* **143**, 291.

Flewellyn, E. H., Nelson, T. E., Jones, W. P., Aren, J. F. and Wagner, D. L. (1983). *Anesthesiology* **59**, 275.

Griffin, J. P. (1984). *35th Annual Refresher Course Lectures of the ASA*. Chicago, Illinois **117**, 1.

Guyton, A. C. (1986). *Textbook of Medical Physiology*, 7th edn. p. 120. Philadelphia: Saunders.

Keith, I. C., Clark, A. G. and Saint John, M. B. (1989). *Canadian Journal of Anaesthesia* **36**, 402.

Kortz, G. (1989). *Seminars in Veterinary Medicine and Surgery (Small Animal)* **4**, 141.

Krone, A., Reuther, P. and Fuhrmeister, U. (1983). *Journal of Neurology* **230**, 111.

LeCouteur, R. A., Dow, S. W. and Sisson, A. F. (1989). *Seminars in Veterinary Medicine and Surgery (Small Animal)* **4**, 146.

Luttgen, P. J. (1989). *Seminars in Veterinary Medicine and Surgery (Small Animal)* **4**, 168.

McGrath, C. J., Rempel, W. E., Jessen, C. R., Addis, P. B. and Crimi, A. J. (1980). *Laboratory Animal Science* **30**, 992.

McGrath, C. J., Rempel, W. E., Addis, P. B. and Crimi, A. J. (1981). *American Journal of Veterinary Research* **42**, 195.

McLeod, M. E. and Creighton, R. E. (1986). *Journal of Child Neurology* **1**, 189.

Mitchell, M. M., Ali, H. H. and Savarese, J. J. (1978). *Anesthesiology* **49**, 44.

Moore, P. and James, O. (1981). *Critical Care Medicine* **9**, 549.

O'Brien, P. J., Cribb, P. J., White, R. J., Olfert, E. D. and Steiss, J. E. (1983). *Canadian Veterinary Journal* **24**, 172.

Pandit, S. K., Kothary, S. P. and Cohen, P. J. (1979). *Anesthesiology* **50**, 156.

Pollard, B. J., Harper, N. J. N. and Doran, B. R. H. (1989). *British Journal of Anaesthesia* **62**, 95.

Ravin, M., Newmark, Z. and Saviello, G. (1975). *Anesthesia and Analgesia* **54**, 216.

Rosenfeld, B., Borel, C. and Hanley, D. (1986). *Archives of Neurology* **43**, 1194.

Seeler, D. C., Dodman, N. H., Norman, W. and Court, M. (1988). *British Veterinary Journal* **144**, 108.

Sharp, N. J. H., Kornegay, J. N. and Lane, S. B. (1989). *Seminars in Veterinary Medicine and Surgery (Small Animal)* **4**, 133.

Shelton, G. D. (1989). *Seminars in Veterinary Medicine and Surgery (Small Animal)* **4**, 126.

Smith, C. E., Donati, F. and Bevan, D. R. (1989). *Canadian Journal of Anaesthesia* **36**, 402.

Smith, M. O. (1989). *Seminars in Veterinary Medicine and Surgery (Small Animal)* **4**, 156.

Index

abdominal trauma 45–6
acepromazine 124
  in cardiac trauma 45
  as cause of bradycardia 95
  in diabetes mellitus 165
  in gastrointestinal disease 151–2
  in geriatric patients 24
  in hyperthyroidism 184
  in hypothyroidism 181
  in liver disease 136
  in myasthenia gravis 230
  in myopathy 234
  in peripheral neuropathy 223
  in phaeochromocytoma 178–9
  problems of 6
  in respiratory disease 60
  in seizures 198
  in spinal cord injury 216
  in trauma 39
acetazolamide 197
acetylcholinesterase 223
acetylprocainamide 115
Addison's disease 170
adrenal cortex, diseases of 170–6
adrenal exhaustion 22
adrenal glands, changes in geriatric
    patients 22–3
adrenal medulla, diseases of 177–80
adrenaline 23, 121–2
adrenergic antagonists 124
α-adrenoceptor antagonists 35
alanine aminotransferase 21, 134, 183
aldosterone 22
alkaline phosphatase 21, 183
aminogluthemide 176
aminophylline 60
amiodarone hydrochloride 119
amputation, forelimb 12
amrinone 128–9
anaesthesia record form 5

anaesthetic drug disposition 38–9
anaesthetic record 3, 11
anaesthetic risk, classification 2
anticholinergics 73
anticholinesterase 85
antidysrhythmic agents 111–21
  Class 1 111–13
  Class 1(a) 114–16
  Class 1(b) 116–17
  Class 2 113–14, 117–18
  Class 3 114, 118–19
  Class 4 114, 119–20
antihistamines 60
aortic stenosis 72, 74–5
aprinidine 117
arginase 134
artificial pancreas 169
aspartate aminotransferase 183
asthma, bronchial 60
ataractics 26
atipamezole 6
atracurium
  in cardiac disease 85
  in liver disease 140
  in myasthenia gravis 231
  in myopathy 235
  in phaeochromocytoma 178
  in renal disease 147
  in respiratory disease 64
  in trauma 41
atrial automaticity, disturbances 92–9
atrial flutter 97–9
atrial premature beats 96–7
atrial septal defects 72
atrioventricular blocks 103–5
atropine sulphate 96, 124–5
  administration with butorphanol 25
  cause of bradycardia 4, 7, 9
  in cardiac disease 73, 82
  in gastrointestinal disease 152

239